Prais

'Incredibly nuanced … So much book … I recommend everybo obviously a huge point of conve these magic pills, and this is the book to read on it' Steven Bartlett, *Diary of a CEO* podcast

'A brilliant synthesis of so much important information' Stephen Fry

'I read this book in four days, and the whole time I have been quoting chunks of it to anyone that will listen. It is a game changer – for all of us. It is balanced and shocking, vitally important and crucially non-judgemental' Davina McCall

'A brilliant book by a master storyteller … Whether you are excited about these drugs or sceptical of them, you will learn so much in *Magic Pill* – it is a must-read' Philippa Perry

'Hari is excellent on the booming ultra-processed food industry and the science of addiction that drives it' *Telegraph*

'[Hari's] own story helps him explore the complexities and wider politics of Ozempic in a nuanced, non-judgemental way. He understands, instinctively, that food culture and body weight are inherently emotional issues, and that we cannot understand rising rates of obesity, or the rise of Ozempic, with reference to health and science alone' *New Statesman*

'I couldn't put *Magic Pill* down. Hari bares his soul about his personal battles with weight … Unlike much of the commentary on this topic, which focuses on short-term problems, such as the drugs' high cost, Hari gets that, in time, they could have as big an impact as the arrival of antidepressants, speculating how they may reshape global health. I found it a fascinating read' *New Scientist*

'Hari gives us a crash course on the new weight loss drugs that will soon be transforming bodies, minds and societies on a massive scale. I had no idea of the power of these drugs, or of the complex web of risks and benefits, until Hari laid it all out with his wonderful technique of saying, "Come on a journey with me as I take these drugs myself while talking with scientists and colourful characters all over the world!"' Jonathan Haidt

'[Hari's] descriptions of his own battles with his weight and yo-yo dieting are both funny and insightful' *Daily Mail*

'Hari marshals his trademark talents at meticulous research, incisive prose, telling anecdote and keen insight to dissect yet another of our dysfunctional culture's troubling features: the obesity epidemic of the past few decades and its treatments. Entertaining without trivialising and deeply informative without being prescriptive, this book leaves us with much to ponder, both on the individual and social levels' Gabor Maté

'A fascinating exploration of weight-loss pharmaceuticals that will redefine our approach to obesity ... This book is not just a personal story, but an examination of how these drugs interact with social norms and personal health, promising liberation – and new psychological dilemmas. As we stand on the brink of a medical revolution, *Magic Pill* is a vital guide through the complex scientific, emotional and cultural landscape of this new frontier' Charles Duhigg

'A fast-paced and fascinating dive into an extremely sensitive topic, written by a charismatic and compulsively readable author' Dan Harris

'Hari unleashes his characteristic blend of personal stories, expert interviews and masterful storytelling to outline the rise of the latest weight loss pharmaceutical ... An easy-to-read and engaging overview of the current weight loss drug landscape' Dr Richard Armitage, *British Journal of General Practice*

'Compelling, thoughtful and fascinating, a revealing and inspiring meditation on weight loss, addiction and the new drugs that may change the way we think about and treat obesity' Maia Szalavitz

'With the intense interest in the new miracle weight loss drugs, we need a balanced look at their promise and peril. Entertaining and highly readable, Johann Hari's *Magic Pill* delivers the information people need to help make a medical decision that might change their future' Arthur C. Brooks

'A deep-dive into Ozempic couldn't be more timely – and necessary' Andy Cohen

'*Magic Pill* may be the most revolutionary, honest and important book you read about weight loss, the body and food. As is always the case with a Johann Hari book, what appears to be a story about the drug, Ozempic, turns out to be a portal into the deepest investigation and revelation on how to live a healthy life' V (formerly Eve Ensler)

JOHANN HARI is the author of three previous internationally bestselling books, translated into 40 languages. His TED talks have been viewed over 90 million times, and his work has been praised by a broad range of people, from Oprah to Noam Chomsky to Joe Rogan. He was also the executive producer of an Oscar-nominated film, and an eight-part TV series with Samuel L. Jackson.

@johannhari101

BY THE SAME AUTHOR

Stolen Focus: Why You Can't Pay Attention – and How To Think Deeply Again

Lost Connections: Uncovering the Real Causes of Depression – and the Unexpected Solutions

Chasing the Scream: The First and Last Days of the War on Drugs

God Save the Queen? The Truth About the Windsors

JOHANN HARI

Magic Pill

A Journey Into the World of the New Weight Loss Drugs

BLOOMSBURY PUBLISHING
LONDON • OXFORD • NEW YORK • NEW DELHI • SYDNEY

BLOOMSBURY PUBLISHING
Bloomsbury Publishing Plc
50 Bedford Square, London, WC1B 3DP, UK
Bloomsbury Publishing Ireland Limited,
29 Earlsfort Terrace, Dublin 2, D02 AY28, Ireland

First published in Great Britain 2024
This edition published 2025

Some names and details of individuals have been changed to preserve their anonymity

A catalogue record for this book is available from the British Library

ISBN: HB: 978-1-5266-7015-1; TPB: 978-1-5266-7014-4;
WATERSTONES SIGNED EDITION: 978-1-5266-8102-7;
PB: 978-1-5266-7016-8; EBOOK; 978-1-5266-7013-7;
EPDF: 978-1-5266-7012-0

2 4 6 8 10 9 7 5 3 1

Typeset by Newgen KnowledgeWorks Pvt. Ltd., Chennai, India
Printed and bound in Great Britain by Clays Ltd, Elcograf S.p.A.

MIX
Paper | Supporting responsible forestry
FSC www.fsc.org
FSC® C018072

To find out more about our authors and books visit www.bloomsbury.com and sign up for our newsletters
For product safety related questions contact productsafety@bloomsbury.com

To the two wisest women I know, V (formerly known as Eve Ensler) and Dorothy Byrne

CONTENTS

CONCLUSION

Introduction
The Holy Grail

In the winter of 2022, the global pandemic seemed to be finally receding, so for the first time in two years, I went to a party. I felt schlubby and slightly self-conscious, because I had gained a stone and a half since the world shut down. Some people say the main reason they survived the pandemic was the vaccine; for me, it was Uber Eats. The party was being thrown by an Oscar-winning actor, and while I didn't expect Hollywood stars to have pudged out as much as the rest of us, I thought there would be a little swelling at the edges.

As I milled around, I felt disconcerted. It wasn't just that nobody had gained weight. They were gaunt. Their cheekbones were higher, their stomachs tighter. This hadn't only happened to the actors. The middle-aged TV executives, the actors' spouses and kids, the agents – everyone I hadn't seen for a few years suddenly looked like their own Snapchat filter, clearer and leaner and sharper.

I bumped into an old friend and said to her, in a kind of shamed mumble, that I guessed everyone really did take up Pilates in lockdown. She laughed. Then, when I didn't laugh back, she stared at me. 'You know it wasn't Pilates, don't you?' I looked back, puzzled, and she said: 'Do you really not know?'

Standing at the side of the dance floor, she pulled up an image on her phone.

I squinted at it in the darkness, as the shrunken partiers all around us shook their bony behinds and discreetly declined the canapés.

On the screen, I could see a light blue plastic tube, with a tiny needle sticking out of it.

~

Later, I would wonder if I had been waiting for that moment all my life.

One afternoon just before Christmas in 2009, I went to my local branch of KFC in east London. I gave my standard order – a bucket of grease and gristle so huge that I'm too embarrassed to list its contents here. The man behind the counter said: 'Johann! We have something for you.' He walked off behind where they fry the chicken, and returned with all the other staff who were working that day. Together, they handed me a massive Christmas card. I opened it. They had addressed it 'To our best customer', and all written personal messages.

My heart sank, because I thought: This isn't even the fried chicken shop I come to the most.

~

Later still, I would wonder if our culture had been waiting for that moment for more than two thousand years.

I learned from the eating disorders expert Hilde Bruch that in ancient Greece, people believed that there had once been a drug that made it possible for people to stay slim, but somewhere along the way the secret formula was lost, never to be found again. Ever since, humans have tried to make this dream a reality – to find a way to hack our biology and reverse weight gain. The headline 'NEW MIRACLE WEIGHT-LOSS DRUG' is as old as headlines themselves.

But when I spoke to experts on obesity across the world, they told me that this time, with this drug, something really was different. Rigorous scientific studies have shown that there is a new generation of drugs – working in a completely new way – that cause the people who use them to lose between 5 and 24 per cent of their body weight. I was told by Tim Spector, a professor of genetic epidemiology at King's College London, that for people with severe obesity: 'It is the Holy Grail that people have been seeking.' Dr Clemence Blouet, an obesity researcher at Cambridge University, said: 'It's the first time we have a safe anti-obesity drug,' and now that the code has been cracked, the discoveries about how to make them better and more effective 'are super-fast' and 'every day there is something new'. Emily Field, a sober-minded analyst at Barclays Bank who studied the likely value of these drugs for investors, wrote a report explaining that she believed the impact these drugs would have on society was comparable to the invention of the smartphone.

This scientific excitement has caused a stampede. In one survey, 47 per cent of Americans said they were willing to pay to take these drugs. Graham MacGregor, who is a professor of cardiovascular medicine at Queen Mary University in London, told me that in Britain, 'within ten years, 20 or 30 per cent of the population will be on obesity drugs ... There's no argument about it.' Some financial analysts believe that the market for them could be worth as much as $200 billion globally by 2030. As a result, Novo Nordisk – the Danish corporation that manufactures one of these drugs, Ozempic – has in one fell swoop become the most valuable company in Europe.

Ozempic and its successors look set to become one of the iconic and defining drugs of our time, on a par with the contraceptive pill and Prozac.

~

Standing on that dance floor, I couldn't remember ever feeling so immediately and intensely conflicted about a topic.

Skimming the basic facts about these drugs on my phone, I realised at once that I could make a passionate case for taking them. The calculations for the exact number of people killed by obesity and poor diet vary. The lowest credible calculation for the US is that it ends 112,000 lives a year – which is more than double the number of people killed in all murders, suicides and accidents involving guns combined. At the upper end, Jerold Mande – an adjunct professor of nutrition at Harvard best known for designing the nutritional label displayed on all food in the United States – warns that 'food-caused illnesses' are estimated to kill 678,000 people every year. He told me this is 'far and away the leading cause of death.'

Here, then, was a chance to finally interrupt our relationship with bad food, and transform it. Nothing else we have tried has worked. We have been serially starving ourselves on diets for decades, and even the most optimistic studies find that only approximately 20 per cent of us succeed at keeping off the weight we lose after a year. Doctors warn us that obesity contributes to 200 known diseases and complications, and explain that we are eating ourselves to death – and we nod gravely, and open the KFC app. Many of us argue for taking on the power of the food companies to stop them from producing ever more addictive junk, but even a figure as popular and charismatic as Michelle Obama couldn't get any traction for that cause.

The proponents of the new weight-loss drugs say this fog of despair is finally parting. Obesity is a biological problem, and now, at last, we have a biological solution. Here is a moment of liberation from a crushing condition which according to some studies doubles your risk of dying when you are older. Here is an opportunity to massively slash the resulting rates of diabetes, dementia and cancer that every major public health body in the world warns about. Here is a drug that could give millions of people back a shot at life.

I could see the power of these arguments. I felt their force. So why was I so uneasy?

I had several huge doubts right away.

In 1960, when my parents were teenagers, they knew almost no obese people. There had been no obese kids at their schools, and hardly any obese adults lived near them. Today, in the two countries where I spend most of my time, obesity levels for adults have hit 26 per cent in Britain and 42.5 per cent in the United States. This transformation – unprecedented in human history – didn't happen because we all contracted a disease. It didn't happen because something went wrong in our biology. It happened because something went disastrously wrong with our society. The food-supply system transformed beyond all recognition. We began to eat foods that didn't exist before – designed by the food industry to be maximally addictive, pumped full of just the right proportions of sugar and salt and starch to keep us chomping. We built cities that it's often impossible to walk or bike around. We became much more stressed, making us seek out more comfort food.

From this perspective, Ozempic and the drugs that have followed represent a moment of madness. We built a food system that poisons us – and then, to keep us away from the avalanche of bad food, we decided to inject ourselves with a different potential poison, one that puts us off all food.

We have started to take these drugs knowing surprisingly little about them. We have no idea about their long-term effects when they are used to treat obesity. We don't know if they will even carry on working for obese people beyond a few years. And chillingly, the scientists who helped create them – as I was going to learn – are not yet sure why they work, or precisely what they are doing to us.

I had another anxiety. We seemed to be finally reaching a moment in our culture where we were learning to stop punishing our bodies and start accepting them, even if they were outside the narrow Western beauty norm. Was this going to slam all that into reverse? Was body positivity going to drown in a tide of Ozempic and its competitor Mounjaro?

Worse than that, what would happen when people with eating disorders get hold of these drugs? What would transpire when we give people determined to starve themselves an unprecedentedly powerful tool to amputate their appetite?

Surrounded by people whose veins were coursing with this drug, I was full of uncertainty, see-sawing between support and scepticism. If we really are about to begin taking drugs that cause sustained massive weight loss, what will that mean – for our personal lives, our health and our societies? Can these drugs really be what they claim? Do they mean we are giving up on challenging the food industry and how it has screwed us over? Do they mean we are giving up on accepting ourselves as we are?

I realised there was one person who I most wanted to discuss all this with. It was because of her that I decided to write this book.

To understand everything that happened next, I need to tell you about Hannah.

~

When I was nineteen years old, I went to the National Student Drama Festival in the faded English seaside town of Scarborough. Every year, students in Britain who've staged plays apply to take part, and theatre professionals come and assess your work, and if it's good enough, you are invited to perform your play by the sea and compete against other students from all over the country, get seen by agents, and potentially win awards. That year, some of my friends got through to the finals, and I went along for the ride. It meant that I watched about twenty plays in a few days. Some were brilliant, and some were lousy, but it was seeing the worst of them all that, in a strange way, changed my life.

One afternoon, I sat down to watch a play called *Atlantica*. It was written and performed as a realistic drama about a group of scientists who were confronting a peculiar and disturbing problem. All over the world, whales were hurling themselves onto beaches and slowly dying. Nobody knew why. It was almost as though these giant blubbery creatures were killing themselves. Were they trying to escape pollution? Did they have a brain disease? What was happening? The play followed these scientists as they took boats out onto the ocean and observed the whales in the wild, to try to figure out this mystery. But when they did, something disturbing happened. Suddenly, the whales charged their boats, trying to break them in half. As the scientists tried to speed away, one cried: 'Oh my God! We've got a sperm whale riding shotgun!'

One of the scientists turned to another and said: 'David – do you think the whales are' (dramatic pause) '*evil*?' Everyone sitting in the audience near us seemed to be leaning into the seriousness of the drama, caught up in its spell. Everyone, that is, except for me – and one other person. In the seat next to mine, in the darkness, there was a young woman who I could see was physically shaking with laughter. I tried really hard not to look at her, because I was afraid I would let out a howl. The more intently the rest of the audience followed the play, the more we began to shake. 'These whales are going to – kill us all!' one of the scientists cried.

Then came the twist. The scientists figured out why the whales were beaching themselves en masse. It turned out they had been watching humanity for some time, and they had concluded that human beings had forgotten how to play. They were tossing themselves onto the world's beaches to urge us to join them in the ocean, to learn how to frolic once again. After explaining this, the lead scientist said: 'There's only one solution.'

The other scientists gasped. 'No,' they said, 'you can't.'

'I have to. I have to – become a whale.' And then, with orchestral music swelling in the background, he leapt into the water and transformed into a whale. Curtain. Applause.

The woman who'd been rocking with suppressed laughter in the darkness hurried out of the auditorium and ran round a corner. I followed her and, without saying a word, we both began to cry laughing. She yelled 'Do you think the whales are … evil?' and I shouted back: 'I have to become – a whale.' I literally fell to the floor.

That night, Hannah and I began to tour the fast-food outlets of Scarborough. We started with a fish and chip shop, then headed to a kebab shop, and then a fried chicken shop. It was only there that I looked at her properly for the first time. She had mousy brown hair and a huge stomach, and she spoke with a musical lilt, as if she was always trying to caress more humour out of the world. At the time, I was overweight, and she liked to describe herself as 'deliciously enormous'.

Right away, we developed our first running joke. We would go into the skeeziest greasy spoon and immediately begin to review it like it was a Michelin-starred restaurant. She took a tiny nibble of a grease-laden kebab and said: 'It's a delightful *amuse-bouche* with … yes –' she chewed some more – 'a deliciously *bold* aftertaste.' We became connoisseurs of grease, sommeliers of Big Mac sauce. We drew up a plan to create our own Michelin stars, except these would be given out by the Michelin Man himself, and the award would be for giving you bigger and bigger tyres around your stomach. As we ate our third kebab, she began to improvise stories about famous suicides who turned out – in a stunning twist – to have been whales. Socrates whale, slugging hemlock rather than face a blubbery tribunal. Sylvia Plath whale, ramming its head into an oven. Virginia Woolf whale, filling its spout with stones and hopping onto land.

As I got to know Hannah, I discovered some hint of why she had developed her stabbingly dark sense of humour. Her grandmother was Jewish and had escaped Germany just in time in the 1930s, and Hannah volunteered at a centre for Holocaust survivors in north London. For years, her social group consisted largely of people who had been in concentration camps. I became friends with one of the survivors she introduced me to, a woman named Trude Levi who had collapsed on her twenty-first birthday on one of the death marches. Hannah liked to say that it's not a coincidence that the Jews and the Irish had both the most horrific histories in Europe and the best sense of humour. You laugh in order to survive. You joke to endure. One of her heroes was Joan Rivers, the outrageous comedian who, after her husband's suicide, went onstage and said as an opening line: 'My husband killed himself and it's my fault. I knew I shouldn't have taken that paper bag off my head while he was fucking me.'

For years, Hannah and I would go to the Edinburgh Festival, a cultural volcano where tens of thousands of performers descend on the medieval streets of the city and perform for over a million annual visitors. You walk up the Royal Mile – the city's central artery – and all around you, people are performing parts of their plays: they're juggling, they're dancing, they're handing you flyers. Inspired by *Atlantica*, we would deliberately seek out the worst-sounding plays and see them all. *Graham – The World's Fastest Blind Man*, a musical about a blind sprinter? We dashed there as fast as our bulk would let us. Every afternoon, we drank milkshakes at the Filling Station, a restaurant on the Royal Mile. Hannah had an incredibly beguiling way of befriending people; she drew them to her with a mixture of extreme vulnerability and extreme vulgarity. Most of her running jokes are so extreme I can't write them down, even here. But I can tell you that one day, one of the waitresses in the Filling Station laughed so hard at one of her obscene jokes that she spilled a banana milkshake all over me.

One evening, an American actor told us about a place I had never heard of. In the US, he said, there is a restaurant named the Heart Attack Grill. At the entrance, there is a huge set of cattle scales, and if you are over 350 pounds (twenty-five stone), you eat for free. As soon as you walk through the door, you have to sign a waiver saying that if the food gives you a heart attack, the responsibility lies entirely with you. You then put on a hospital gown, and you are served by waitresses dressed as nurses. If you don't finish all of the massive portions of food, they spank you with a paddle. We immediately promised ourselves that one day we would go there and toast our friendship in banana milkshake.

Hannah liked to talk to men in public places in startlingly frank sexual ways. She enjoyed seeing the shock on people's faces, as if she was refusing to be ashamed of her weight and her body, and defying the world to take her as she was. Her voice had a soothing, mellifluous quality that often jarred with the things she said – she once told me she wanted people hearing her to feel like they were listening to a children's TV host gently reading out the words of Charles Manson.

And yet, existing alongside this spirit of joy and play, she would show sudden bursts of being terribly afraid. She would have panic attacks, seemingly out of nowhere. She hated getting on public transport. She took a very high dose of antidepressants. She was convinced that politics could turn very dark, very fast, that the stability we lived through would turn out to be an illusion, and the world would turn out to be a charnel house, so our job was to amuse ourselves as best we could before it consumed us. (On 7th July 2005, after a terrorist attack on the London Underground, she immediately texted me: 'Now you see why I am a taxi person.') She had a level of fear appropriate to the Holocaust survivors she volunteered with, not to a person who had grown up in 1980s and 90s Britain. She always had the vigilance of somebody who was ready to run.

We never talked about why she ate so much, except through our obsessive surreal joshing. I never heard her express any concern about her weight. We once watched a documentary about a person so obese that they had to dismantle his house to get him out for medical treatment. She said: 'I have a new life goal.'

Our friendship became a rat-a-tat-tat of shared jokes and shared obsessions. We loved Stephen Sondheim musicals, and we prided ourselves that our favourite was, at that time, the most obscure: *Merrily We Roll Along*. It's the story of three friends, told backwards: it starts with the central characters as jaded, bitter, drunk forty-somethings, and then rolls back the years, scene after scene, until they are young and naive and optimistic, just starting out. There's a song in it – 'Old Friends' – about how, even if you argue with your old friends, they're always there, lodestars for how you live. I thought of it as my and Hannah's song.

But then something happened. Every time I met her, it struck me anew that Hannah was one of the cleverest people I've ever known, constantly coming up with brilliant ideas out of thin air. For example, the day the United States invaded Afghanistan, she started improvising, over dinner, a novel about an undercover US agent in Kabul, written in the style of Raymond Chandler. I can still remember the first line: 'She wore her burkas tight, and her morals loose.' I urged her to write it all down, and to translate her brilliance onto the page. I was starting to become successful as a journalist, but she was just staying at home a lot of the time, feeling anxious, not working. It seemed to me that Hannah had chosen to stay hidden. I kept pressing her to do more, and as I pushed her, she retreated. We began to argue. I was pushing her to be everything I felt she could be. Thinking about it now, perhaps she thought I was judging and condemning her.

As we quarrelled, I became increasingly frustrated. Every flash of genius I saw in her seemed even more like a waste. Why was this being confined only to me and her small group of friends? Why scatter it to the wind?

Somewhere along the way, this dynamic meant we pushed each other away. The last night I remember seeing her was in 2008, when we watched Barack Obama's victory at a big party in my apartment. But even as the gap since we'd last seen each other yawned wider, I was always sure we would meet up again somewhere down the road. We had too many shared jokes, I believed, for our bond to break. Often, I would hear something funny and think – I must phone Hannah and tell her that. In my mind, she was somewhere hailing a taxi, milkshake in hand, laughing, always laughing.

Then, one morning, in early 2021, I received a phone call. Hannah's family had posted on Facebook that she had died. In the days that followed, I called our mutual friends who were still in touch with her. They told me what they knew. Several years before, she had developed severe back pain, and started taking opioid-based painkillers. She became addicted, and found it really hard to stop, but she managed to do it. Then she developed type 2 diabetes. Then she developed cancer, and felt that taking opioids would constitute a relapse, so she went through the gruelling treatment in agony. She was weakened by the cancer but survived. Then she got Covid, and was weakened some more, but survived again. Then one night, she began to choke while eating and went into cardiac arrest.

I was incredulous that somebody who took such joy in living could have died in her mid-forties. I kept running over her old jokes in my mind, writing down as many as I could, as if they were slipping away from me. I felt desperately sad that she didn't reach out to me when she was ill. She must have thought that I would judge her, or that I wouldn't show up at all.

The heart of our shared sense of humour was our love of bad food, and our commitment to consuming it in epic quantities. I felt queasy as I thought about that now. It's possible for anyone, no matter what their weight, to choke and for their heart to suddenly fail. But it seemed very likely that her obesity had caused her death. She was weakened by a series of illnesses, and obesity makes it more likely you will get cancer, more likely you will become seriously sick with Covid, and more likely your heart will fail when faced with a stressful event. I also strongly suspect that the way she compulsively ate and crammed huge amounts of food into her mouth may have contributed to her choking.

I looked at the remembered jokes I had written down, and wanted to laugh at them one more time, but now they turned to dust in my mouth.

Not long afterwards, I was in Las Vegas, researching a different book. I decided to keep my promise to her and go to the Heart Attack Grill, to toast our friendship in banana milkshake. I stood by the entrance and watched people standing on the cattle scales, hoping to clock in at higher than 350 pounds so they could eat for free. I saw the waitresses dressed as nurses, spanking people who didn't finish their giant servings of fries. I gazed over the people wolfing down massive burgers, and buckets of milkshake, and onion rings the size of a whole plate.

I couldn't bring myself to go in. It felt like the joke was, in the end, on us.

~

Joseph Stalin reputedly said that one death is a tragedy but a million deaths is just a statistic. I guess I had known since I was a teenager that the major scientific bodies in the world warn that obesity kills large numbers of people every year – but in my twenties and thirties, it had seemed like an abstraction. Now Hannah had left a hole in the world. I am certain that nobody in my life will ever again be able to reduce me to the helpless, hysterical laughter of childhood as much as she did.

Hannah's death should have been a warning sign to me. As a child, I ate almost nothing but junk and processed food, but my weight only started to blow up in my late teens, when I began taking chemical antidepressants. Since then my weight had yo-yoed between being slightly underweight to quite seriously obese, with a waistline that ranged from 30 inches to 40 inches.

By the time the pandemic was dissipating, I was creeping back into the danger zone. I am five foot eight and I weighed fourteen and a half stone – a BMI just over 30, which was bad, but my other indicators were worse. When my trainer at the gym tested to see what percentage of my body was fat, he winced at the score: 32 per cent. 'If I was a sandwich, you wouldn't want to eat me,' I said with a weak smile. Later I googled and learned that the most blubbery mammal in the animal kingdom, the whale, has 35 per cent body fat.

I knew that for me in particular, this condition wasn't safe. My grandfather died of a heart attack when he was the age I am now, forty-four. My uncle died in his sixties of a heart attack. My father developed diabetes and had to have a quadruple heart bypass in his early seventies. Worse still, my fat was in the worst possible place for my health. Dr Shauna Levy, an obesity specialist at the Tulane University School of Medicine in New Orleans, told me that if your fat is distributed evenly across your body, that's less harmful to your health than for 'people with central adiposity – skinny arms, skinny legs, big belly. They are more likely to have diabetes and high blood pressure.' But I love life. I want as much of it as possible. I want to be around for a long time. (I can hear in my mind how Hannah would respond to all this. 'Do you really think you love life more than you love Big Mac sauce?')

Many times before, I had received wake-up calls about weight that didn't wake me up. Sometimes a jolt would spur me to cut back on the junk food and exercise more, and the effects could be quite dramatic when I did. I even had a few years when I was at the lower end of the BMI chart, and my cheekbones emerged, like the lost continent of Atlantis from beneath the ocean. But I always slid back sooner or later, feeling slumped and ashamed. It's true I was nowhere near as obese as Hannah, but I suspect I had a larger genetic risk for cardiovascular problems than her.

For all my obvious doubts about Ozempic, I also wondered: Could this possibly be the way to break some of the danger that my own health was in? I learned that several people I knew were already taking the drug. The men would admit it quite freely, while the women would offer long stories about intermittent fasting or a fantastic new spa, and then quietly concede that, yes, they were on it too. I could see weight was falling off them, and their doctors were telling them that all their key indicators of health were dramatically improving.

I was full of doubt – about my weight, and these drugs, and about the future. But I kept thinking of Hannah. I would lie awake at night and punch her number into my phone. We became friends just before mobile phones became widespread, so she had the last phone number I ever committed to memory. I would think of all the things I wanted to say to her – the jokes I'd heard, the regrets I wanted to offer.

Then, quite abruptly, I decided that I should start to take these drugs. It was a snap decision, and later I realised I was driven by impulses I didn't fully understand at the time. I went to see a private doctor, and after some brief questions and some cursory measuring, he agreed to give me Ozempic. A few days later, a courier arrived at my home bearing a white parcel. I was too nervous to open it on my own, so I waited for a friend's party the next night, and we tore it open as a group. Inside, there was a fat blue pen and some tiny white needles. I hate syringes – I'm the kind of wuss who has to look away and sing to myself during blood tests. But this needle was tiny. The instructions said that once a week, all I had to do was twist the teeny needle onto the end of the pen, poke it into my stomach, and push down on the base of the pen to let it flow into my bloodstream.

When I stabbed my flab with it, I felt very little – a sting no worse than an insect bite. I heard only the click-click-click coming from the pen as the drug was released. The Ozempic began to flow through my body for the first time.

I know a few people who have had near-death experiences, and they say that their lives really did flash before their eyes. In that moment, it happened with my culinary life. I pictured all the foods I have gorged on since I was a kid. I saw in my mind the mushrooms and bright yellow bananas made out of sugar that I would stuff into my mouth at the age of five. I thought of salt and vinegar chipsticks, a kind of sticky potato chip popular in the 1980s. I pictured more KFC than Colonel Sanders could conjure in his wildest, wettest dream.

I pictured the hundreds of branches of McDonald's I had sought out all over the world, like a plastic womb I could always retreat to wherever I found myself. I saw the lowest McDonald's in the world, by the Dead Sea in Israel. I saw the first ever McDonald's in Russia, a symbol of Western freedom that shut down shortly after I visited because of the invasion of Ukraine. I saw the branch of McDonald's I most love, at the end of the Strip in Las Vegas, just beyond the Luxor, where the customers are all either tourists who got lost or homeless people who live in the tunnels beneath the city. I saw the scariest McDonald's I ever visited, in El Salvador, where there was a guard on the door holding a huge machete. I asked him why he had that weapon and he said it was because the authorities had taken away their machine guns. There are 38,000 branches of McDonald's in the world, and I felt like I could see them all before me, slowly fading away.

I stood up and rubbed the spot where the needle had been. I felt nothing.

It seemed like a bizarre moment in history – when nearly half of us would be keen to inject ourselves with a drug to stop us from wanting to eat. I wondered: How did I get here? More importantly, how did *we* get here?

~

To understand what these drugs will mean for us all, I went on a journey around the world, where I interviewed over a hundred experts and other people who have been affected by these questions. I got to know some of the key scientists who developed these drugs, and also their biggest critics. I followed the trail of this science to some strange and unexpected places, from a stadium filled with trampolining teens in Iceland, to a diet expert who watched me eat a cinnamon bun in Minneapolis, to a restaurant serving poisonous fish in Tokyo.

What I learned is complex. If you want a book uncritically championing these drugs, or alternatively a book damning them, I am afraid I can't give it to you. The more you look at this topic, and the wider debate about obesity, the more complicated it gets. When it comes to food and diet, we crave simple solutions, but this is a topic fraught with complexity, with question marks at every turn. I started this journey full of doubt, and I finished it knowing much more, but still riven with uncertainty. I hope, in the end, this is a strength. One of my favourite writers, Graham Greene, said, 'When we are not sure, we are alive.' I felt strangely alive while working on this book. The truth is that there are huge potential benefits to these drugs and huge potential risks, and everyone reading this book will weigh those differently. My hope is that we can find our way through the complexity together.

If we do, we can see that these drugs reframe – and to some degree may even resolve – some of the oldest and hoariest debates about obesity. Why have we gained so much weight in the last forty years? What really causes weight gain? Is losing weight a matter of willpower? How should we think about our bodies?

I want to make you aware, right at the start, of a few caveats. Firstly, I'm not a scientist: I'm a journalist who was given a rigorous training in the social sciences at Cambridge University. The people I interviewed are experts; I'm not. Secondly, when it comes to these drugs, there's a lot we don't know, and even what we do know is hotly debated. Scientists disagree on even basic aspects of it. This is a mass experiment, carried out on millions of people, and I am one of the guinea pigs. Throughout the book, I'm going to flag up what we can know now, and where the scientists disagree, I'll try to summarise their different perspectives in a sympathetic and respectful way.

Thirdly, the debate about Ozempic and the other weight-loss drugs is made even more complicated by the fact that it is taking place at the same time as a necessary debate about how we can challenge stigma against overweight and obese people. This conversation is so charged that even using the words 'overweight' and 'obese' will upset and anger some people. I hate to upset people who have soaked up so much cruelty directed at them. I have a lot of sympathy with the people making the case for body positivity, and on several crucial points, I think they are right, the science backs them up, and we need to listen to them. But – after giving it a great deal of thought – I do not believe we should stop using these words. The World Health Organization – the leading medical body in the world – defines being overweight or obese as having 'abnormal or excessive fat accumulation that presents a risk to health'. The evidence is overwhelming that this is a real phenomenon: you can harm your health by gaining weight above a certain level. It is as strong as the proof that smoking causes lung cancer. This is why every major medical institution in the world continues to warn about an obesity crisis.

If we give up this language, we lose our ability to describe a crucial part of reality, and although that might provide some temporary psychological relief, in the end it helps nobody. For reasons that will become clear, I believe you can both oppose the vile stigma that is directed at overweight people, and also explain – with love and compassion – the scientific evidence about obesity and why we need solutions to it.

~

At every stage of working on this book, my mind kept coming back to the musical Hannah and I loved, *Merrily We Roll Along*. I thought again of its plot – of how at the start, we meet three friends when they are middle-aged and jaded, and with each scene, the clock runs backwards, and we see them become younger and healthier. In the most optimistic scenario, that is what these drugs seem to offer us. We get to roll back the clock – to a world where people like Hannah get to have a chance at health.

But as I learned, we've had several moments in the past when a new diet drug was hailed as a 'magic pill', and then had to be yanked from the shelves because it was more deadly than obesity itself.

There are three different senses in which these drugs could be a magic pill. The first is in the sense that they could be a solution to this problem – one so swift and so simple that it seems almost miraculous. The second is that they could turn out to be an unintended illusion that, when you look closer, is not what it seems. They might not always work exactly as claimed, or they could come with downsides that are not visible at first glance. Or they could be magic in a third sense. Perhaps one of the most famous stories about magic is the Disney cartoon *Fantasia*. It's a parable about how when you start to unleash an unknown force like magic, it can easily spiral out of your control, and have effects you could never have imagined at the start.

That is why, as I felt the Ozempic course through my veins for the first time, I needed to know: what kind of magic, exactly, is this?

1

Finding the Treasure Chest
How the drugs work

I opened my eyes and immediately felt that something was off. Thwacking my alarm clock into silence, I lay there for five minutes, trying to figure out what it was. It was two days since I had started taking Ozempic. I felt very mildly nauseous, but it was not severe – if it had happened on a normal day, it wouldn't have stopped me from doing anything. So that wasn't it. It took me a while to realise what it was. I always wake up ravenously hungry, but on that morning, I had no appetite at all. It was gone.

I got out of bed and, on autopilot, went through my normal morning routine. I left my flat and went to a local cafe run by a Brazilian woman named Tatiana, where my order is always the same: a large toasted bread roll, filled with chicken and mayonnaise. As I sat there reading the newspapers, the food was placed in front of me, and I looked at it. I felt like I was looking at a block of wood. I took a bite. It tasted fine. Normal. I took three or four more bites, and I felt full. I left almost all of it on the plate. As I hurried out, Tatiana called after me, 'Are you sick?'

I went to my office and wrote for three hours. Normally, by noon, I would have a snack, something small and sugary, and then at about 1 p.m. I would go down the street to a local Turkish cafe for lunch. It got to 2 p.m. and I wasn't hungry. Again, my sense of routine kicked in, and again, I went to the cafe and asked for my standard order, a large Mediterranean lamb with rice and bread. I managed to eat a third of it. It seemed to me for the first time to be incredibly salty, like I was drinking seawater.

I wrote some more, and at 7 p.m. I left my office to go and meet a friend in Camden Market, one of my favourite parts of London. We walked between the stalls, staring at food from every part of the world. Normally, I could stuff my face from three different stalls, but that night, I had no hunger. I couldn't even manage a few mouthfuls. I went home, feeling exhausted, and went to sleep at the unprecedentedly early time of 9 p.m.

As that first week passed, it felt like the shutters had come down on my appetite, and now only tiny peeks of light could get through. I was about 80 per cent less hungry than I normally am. The sense of mild nausea kept stirring and passing. When I got on the bus or in a car, I felt a kind of exaggerated travel sickness. Whenever I ate, I became full startlingly fast. The best way I can describe it is to ask you to imagine that you have just eaten a full Christmas dinner with all the trimmings, and then somebody popped up and offered you a whole new meal to get started on. Some people say Ozempic makes them find food disgusting. To me, it made food, beyond small quantities, feel unfeasible.

On the fifth night, a friend came by to watch a movie, and we flicked through Uber Eats. The app suggested all my usual haunts. I realised I couldn't eat any of this food now. Instead, she got a kebab, and I had a bowl of vegetable soup. On the sixth day, I took my godsons out, and they wanted to go into McDonald's. When they got Happy Meals and I got nothing at all, one of them said suspiciously: 'Who are you and what have you done with Johann Hari?'

I wanted to understand what was happening to my body. I figured that the best people to educate me were the scientists who made the key discoveries that led to the development of Ozempic and the other new weight-loss drugs. So I began to track many of them down and interview them, along with many other key scientists working in the field. Almost all of them have received funding from the pharmaceutical companies that now profit from these drugs, and we should bear that in mind as we hear what they say.

They taught me that these extraordinary effects were coming from manipulating a tiny hormone named GLP-1 that exists in my gut and my brain, and in yours. To understand what it is, I think it helps to understand how it was discovered.

~

One day in 1984, a lean 28-year-old Canadian research scientist walked into a lab in Massachusetts General Hospital and felt instinctively uneasy. Daniel Drucker had been assigned to work in one of the huge buildings there, and he expected to find a shiny state-of-the-art set-up. Instead, it was shabby and run-down. As he sat at his bench, pigeons were constantly cooing from their nests in the roof above him, threatening to poop and contaminate any experiment he might carry out.

He knew he had only made it to this lab in the first place by a few thin twists of fate. His mother had been born in Poland and fled the Nazis without a moment to spare – the day after she got out of the ghetto, her mother and sister were shot dead. She survived by hiding in attics. Even after she made it to the safety of Canada and learned her relatives had been murdered, she never stopped searching for them. She would ask her son: what if the witnesses who saw them being killed were wrong, and they're still out there alive somewhere, looking for me?

Daniel trained to be a thyroid specialist, so he was surprised and disappointed when the lab's head told him that the hospital didn't have any thyroid work and he was assigned to a different project. Every human body is made up of cells, and in the 1970s, scientists had discovered new tools they could use to figure out for the first time what is going on inside them. They were working their way through many of the cells, and Daniel was allocated the inner workings of something named the glucagon gene. Very little was known about its deeper structure. Go figure it out, he was told.

It didn't particularly excite him, but it was work, so he got started. He found it tough. He told me that when it came to clinical medicine 'I was very capable, but when I got to the lab, I was completely incapable. I had never done [this kind of] research before. It was a struggle for me.' When he successfully carried out an experiment that teased apart the functioning of this particular cell, he was just relieved that 'I actually managed to do something with these clumsy wooden hands', and that the pigeons didn't poop on the results.

As he investigated what was happening inside the glucagon gene, he started to look into a specific question. He knew the gene consisted of different constituent parts – it's a long chain – and one of them, found at the end, was a snippet of the overall genetic code, labelled as GLP-1. Daniel and the other scientists in his team wanted to figure out if this part of the gene was just an inert or redundant bit of code that didn't do anything on its own, or if it could be teased out and investigated as a thing in its own right. After a lot of experimenting, he discovered that, in fact, it could be broken off from the wider code.

Once he knew this could be done, he began to ask: what does GLP-1 actually do? He decided to start putting it into petri dishes, to see how it interacted with many different chemicals that are found in that part of the body.

It was on one of those afternoons that he tried something that, years later, he told me was his 'aha moment' – one that was going to reshape his whole career, and the lives of millions of people, including my own.

When he mixed GLP-1 with some cells that produce insulin, he noticed something striking: the GLP-1 stimulated the creation of insulin. Something about this tiny gut hormone could spur the making of another hormone, one that is essential for your body to regulate your blood sugar levels and keep you alive.

His mind flickered immediately to diabetes, a medical condition where your body doesn't produce enough insulin, leading to all sorts of disastrous health effects. He could see, in the Petri dish right in front of him, that GLP-1 'was making more insulin'. Could it be used to treat diabetics? Another scientist on the team named Svetlana Mojsov worked with a group to put GLP-1 into a rat's pancreas. She found that there, too, it led to the creation of more insulin. This meant it didn't just work in a dish in a lab – it worked in a living creature. Around the same time, a team in Copenhagen put GLP-1 into a pig's pancreas. They found the same effect.

But finding a way to apply this to human diabetics was going to be a long road – and some surreal turns had to take place first.

~

Three thousand miles away from Daniel, in the Hammersmith Hospital in west London, John Wilding was disturbed. He was a young doctor, and one day in the early 1990s, he was told that there was a man he needed to see urgently in the emergency room, who had been brought there in an unusual way. When the paramedics had arrived at the patient's home, they discovered he was so obese that he couldn't get through his own front door. Left with no other option, they had to get firefighters to smash his windows and haul him out using a crane.

John diagnosed that the patient had something called severe obesity hypoventilation, a disorder that sometimes afflicts people who've gained extreme amounts of weight, where they breathe too slowly, so they can't get enough oxygen into their systems. Once he was stabilised, the patient told John that he had an insatiable appetite: he felt he couldn't stop eating, no matter what he did. John watched as the patient ate one pack of sandwiches after another. Not long after, he died of a massive pulmonary embolism.

John was also a research scientist at the hospital, and he was following the early research on GLP-1 keenly. Once Daniel Drucker had identified that the hormone could be separated and have such striking effects, scientists had begun to probe another question. Where and when, they wondered, does GLP-1 get made in the human body?

They discovered something crucial.

After you eat, your GLP-1 levels spike in your gut. They wondered if it was some kind of natural signal, telling you to stop eating. You've had enough. You're full.

So John asked: if GLP-1 is released when you eat, could you reduce a person's appetite by artificially boosting it? He injected GLP-1 into rats, and found that, as John suspected, it had a dramatic impact on their appetites. It was 'a really quite powerful effect', he said. This was the first round of proof that GLP-1 didn't just affect insulin and blood sugar. It seemed to have effects that boosted satiety – the sensation of feeling full.

Now the scientists asked: could GLP-1 be used to help people like John's patient, who had died in such grim circumstances?

The lab investigated more. They injected GLP-1 directly into people, by jabbing them in the gut with a tiny needle. Incredibly, it worked: they felt more full, and they ate less. But there was a problem. GLP-1 spikes in your gut and then disappears very quickly. Within a few minutes, it's washed out of your system. So to get people to eat less, they had to inject them three times a day, and even then, it only stifled their appetites for a short time. It was tantalising, but frustrating. These experiments proved that there was a real effect of GLP-1 on human appetite, but nobody was going to inject themselves three times a day to slightly take the edge off their hunger. Their findings didn't seem to point to anything very practical in the real world.

In the wake of these experiments, the interest in GLP-1 as a potential treatment for obesity began to wane. Instead, research ramped up on other newly discovered gut hormones, which scientists thought might be more useful. It looked like this story was over, and the research into GLP-1 had turned out to be one of the many alleyways in scientific research that come to nothing.

~

Then a breakthrough came from totally out of left field.

After Daniel and the other scientists in their lab published the genetic code of GLP-1, a biochemist in the Bronx named John Eng noticed something weird. It was almost identical to a chemical that he had discovered in the venom of the deadliest lizard in the United States.

The Gila monster is a sluggish, slow-moving beast that slithers across the deserts of Arizona and New Mexico, and grows to be up to twenty-two inches long. If you are brave enough to catch one and extract its venom, you get a copy of GLP-1 – but with a crucial twist. Whereas natural GLP-1 degrades in the human body within minutes, the lizard's venom is stronger and lasts for hours. So if you inject it into a human, you can find out what happens if their GLP-1 levels are elevated over a longer time than could ever happen in nature.

After reading John Eng's research, Daniel Drucker – who was still eager to see if these insights could be used to help diabetics – realised he had to get hold of these monsters, to try it. That was easy to say, but hard to do. They are deadly creatures and the trade in them is tightly regulated. He tried some dodgy-sounding 'lizard-dealers' he found in the phone book in areas where they run wild, but he realised that they couldn't provide the legitimate paperwork he needed to conduct university research on them. In the end, Daniel persuaded a zoo out west to sell him one. 'I was a little ambivalent,' he told me, 'because I kept on saying to the director of the zoo, "You know I'm going to euthanise this animal?" I thought, naively, of zoos as protectors of wildlife. He just said: "250 bucks."' One of Daniel's colleagues flew out to collect the unlucky creature, and stashed the lizard in a bag in the overhead bins on his flight back. When Daniel saw it in his lab, he was struck by how beautiful the animal was.

Thanks to this little desert-dwelling monster, scientists all over the world were able to figure out what happens if the effects of GLP-1 can be made to last. They discovered that the longer GLP-1 – or a copy of it – stays in your body, the more insulin your body makes. So the drug companies started to do something extraordinary. They got better at making copies of GLP-1 that last longer and longer in your system. Suddenly, instead of lasting a few minutes like real GLP-1, or a few hours like the lizard venom, they invented new 'agonists' – or copies – of it that could remain in your system for a whole week before it was broken down. Using the lizard venom and other methods, they created medicines containing these GLP-1 replicas. In 2005, these medicines were approved for use by diabetics, and they quickly began to be used all over the world. It worked. The drugs brought diabetics' blood sugar under greater control, and significantly reduced their problems. 'That was unbelievably exciting,' Daniel said.

It didn't take long for people to notice something else. These diabetics also often lost a huge amount of weight. Nobody had told them to cut back, and they didn't seem to be making major lifestyle changes, yet the pounds were falling off. So back at the Hammersmith Hospital, John Wilding's team wanted to see – if this drug was given to obese people rather than diabetics, would they lose weight too? They got funding from the Danish company Novo Nordisk to investigate.

They faced a big and immediate obstacle. When you give these drugs to people, they often experience nasty side effects at first. The most common is that they feel nauseous, sometimes violently so. This meant the researchers had to build up the dose very slowly. They incrementally increased it over sixteen weeks to get the trial subjects to the target dose of 2.4mg. 'We saw some people losing twenty-five or thirty kilos of weight, which we'd never seen before in clinical trials,' John said. 'We were just really impressed.'

One day in 2021, the executives at Novo Nordisk, from their corporate offices in Copenhagen, gathered together the scientists working in the field on Zoom to announce something historic. They now had the official results of their major trial giving Ozempic to obese people. They had discovered that for people who were in the trial for sixty-eight weeks and were given the real drug, they lost an average of 15 per cent of their body weight, compared to just 2.4 per cent who had been given a placebo.

This meant it was officially the most successful weight-loss drug in history.

'Almost everybody's mouth opened. It's like – wow. Just wow,' Professor Robert Kushner, who carried out the later stages of the clinical trials, recalled. It was like a moment in a game show, where you realise you've won the jackpot.

He said: '"Game-changer" is what came to mind right away.'

~

A lot was now becoming clear. These gut hormones create the natural signals in your body, telling you to stop eating. Scientists had shown that if you can create a replica of those hormones, blast them into your system, and keep them there for a week, you'll eat much less. But the drug seemed to change more than the patients' bodies. It seemed to change their minds.

Robert told me that previously, the people taking part in the clinical trials had often been obsessed with food. Then, when they were on the drug, 'they will tell you ... "All those foods that I had cravings for and preference for, I don't have much interest in them any more. I'm not thinking about food as much." '

The significance of the fact that it seemed to change how the patients *thought* only became clear later, as you'll see in a future chapter.

~

Several clinical trials also investigated something else that would be hugely significant for people who wanted to use the drug. What happens to you when you stop taking it?

It turns out that after they quit, most people regain two-thirds of the weight they have lost within a year. A spokesperson for Novo Nordisk explained to me that the clinical trials 'demonstrate that weight regain is likely once treatment with Wegovy (the exact same drug as Ozempic marketed with a different name) is stopped. Clinical experts consulted by Novo Nordisk view obesity as a chronic disease that should be managed similar to other long-term health conditions such as diabetes and hypertension.'

This means that for the medication to work, you have to take it for ever. It's not like taking a drug to treat malaria, where you take a course, and then it's done and you're cured. It's like taking statins to lower your cholesterol levels, or blood pressure tablets – you have to keep using it, or lose the effect.

This drug, in other words, isn't a holiday fling. It's a lifelong marriage.

~

Not long after that meeting in Copenhagen, Daniel Drucker – the Canadian scientist who first identified GLP-1 in that dusty pigeon-strewn lab in 1984 – wrote: 'It took almost four decades and thousands of dedicated scientists to slowly change the options for people with type 2 diabetes, cardiovascular disease, and now obesity.' Novo Nordisk now manufactures and markets two forms of semaglutide – Ozempic, for diabetics, and Wegovy, for obese people. They are the same drug, sold for different purposes, and Wegovy can be prescribed at higher doses.

Daniel told me that people often come up to him asking questions about these drugs. When he went to the dentist recently, the hygienist was peppering him with questions about Ozempic, even as his mouth was full of metal and he could barely speak. 'It's awkward for me to go to family parties now. I get buttonholed.' He has a friend at his golf club who's always been a big eater, and Daniel was amazed one day when, out of the blue, he offered to share his pizza with him. In twenty years of friendship, he'd never offered to share any food. The guy turned to his golfing buddies and announced: 'I'm on Drucker's drug. I'm just not hungry any more!'

The scientists involved believe this is just the beginning. In the past few years, researchers working with a different pharmaceutical company, Eli Lilly, began to experiment with a drug named Mounjaro that simulated not just GLP-1 but another gut hormone known as GIP. Incredibly, the people taking this drug lost, on average, 21 per cent of their body weight in the clinical trials. The company has also developed another drug known as 'Triple G', which simulates GLP-1, GIP and a third hormone named glucagon. Early studies suggest it produces 24.2 per cent weight loss. I was told by Robert Kushner, who carried out one of those key stages of the obesity trials of the drugs: 'It's like we finally found the treasure chest – what regulates body weight … Gut hormones.' As a result, there are now more than seventy anti-obesity drugs in development.

Daniel told me that soon there will be no need for injections. 'It's possible in a few years, we'll have pills that you can take once a day that give you hopefully very similar, robust effects. Then, instead of the shots costing hundreds of dollars a month, or thousands of dollars a month if you live in the United States, the pills could cost a dollar to two a day.' In a sign of how fast this story is moving, only a few months after he said this to me, two major studies were published that revealed semaglutide pills – known as Rybelsus – work just as effectively as the injections. Carel Le Roux, a scientist who played a key role in developing these drugs, said: 'When a baby develops, they start by crawling. They're crawling for a long time, and then they just stand up and walk. We're at that inflection point. It's going to be incredible, what happens in the next three years. That's very exciting.'

~

As the drugs began to be used widely across the world, financial analysts started to figure out what this would mean for the global economy. Strategists at Barclays Bank urged investors to move away from the fast-food and snacks markets. There's already been a decline in the value of the stocks of the doughnut company Krispy Kreme, which analysts directly attributed to the growing popularity of Ozempic. Similarly, Mark Schneider, the chief executive of Nestlé, said that 'food and snacking-related categories are the most impacted. In our case that will be the frozen food side of things, confectionery, and to some extent, ice cream.' Morgan Stanley calculated that, because people drink less alcohol when they're on these drugs, there will likely be $3.5 billion knocked out of the market for booze in the US over two years.

The effects are rippling out into unexpected parts of the economy. Companies selling devices for hip and knee replacements have seen their values plunge, because obesity causes so much damage to those parts of the body. An analyst for Jefferies Financial said that airlines are poised to save millions of dollars a year because less jet fuel is burned when you are flying slimmer people. Even jewellers have seen a shift in their business, because people's fingers are shrinking as they shed weight, so they need their wedding rings to be refitted.

~

Throughout my first six months on Ozempic, my friend Danielle was pregnant, and as her pregnancy developed, she would say it was like we were on opposite trajectories. While her belly swelled, mine was shrivelling. I lost a stone and a half. On the BMI chart, I went from obese (marked in a bright red) to the middle of overweight (yellow), and as the months passed and I lost another stone, I got to the upper end of a healthy weight (depicted in a soothing green). My body fat percentage fell from 32 per cent to 22 per cent. It was the fastest and most dramatic weight loss of my life.

I felt lighter and quicker on my feet, and that boosted my confidence enough that I started to strut a little. People began to notice. 'Wow, you're losing weight,' acquaintances said when they saw me in the street. One of my godsons said: 'Hey, Johann, I didn't know you had a neck!' In the third month, my neighbour's hot gardener hit on me and asked for my phone number.

I realised it was exactly what I had wanted, and I was thrilled (especially about the gardener). I had told myself going in that I was concerned primarily about my health – but I now saw that a desire to look better had been a big driver for me all along. I felt genuinely grateful as I interviewed the scientists who'd developed this drug. While they told me about their discoveries, I could literally feel the effects playing out by placing my hand on my stomach. When I was talking with one of the scientists who'd worked on GLP-1 in a cafe in London and listening to her explain the drug's potentially revolutionary effects, I watched people walking past us on the busy street. Most of them had not heard about Ozempic or the other weight-loss drugs yet. Many of them were overweight or obese, and I thought: You don't know what's about to happen. You don't know how this could be about to help you change.

But I was surprised to notice that, at the same time, I also felt disconcerted and out of sorts a lot of the time. I wasn't feeling an urge to recommend Ozempic to other people.

In fact, I felt pensive, and tense. I didn't understand it. I'd got what I wanted – a boost to my health, and a boost to my self-esteem. So why did I still feel so ambivalent about it?

~

At first, I thought it was because of the side effects, which were surprisingly persistent. My nausea, which had been gentle at first, would suddenly surge at random moments and leave me feeling like I was on a boat in the middle of a storm. With Ozempic or Wegovy, everyone starts by taking a dose of 0.25mg a week, then after a month they go up to 0.5mg, and then a month later to a full 1mg. (Some people go to even higher doses after that.)

Every time I increased my dose, I felt significantly worse for at least a week. One evening I found myself dry-heaving next to a pot plant in Zurich airport, while a Swiss woman, who clearly thought I was drunk, gave me dirty looks. This sickness was intermittent, and most of the time I didn't feel it at all, but when it came, it was horrible. It occurred alongside other strange effects. Sometimes I would lie awake at night and find myself uncontrollably burping. At its worst, I was belching up bile and thought I was going to throw up. I also became constipated.

The grimmest side effects for me lay elsewhere. For many people, when they take these drugs, their resting heart rate increases. I would sit reading a book, or lie in bed, and feel my heart racing. My mind often interpreted this as anxiety and would start racing to match my elevated heartbeat. I had to cut back on caffeine to counteract this effect, and even that didn't totally solve the problem – invariably, whenever I increased my dose, I felt anxious for at least a week, and even after that, I felt like I could more easily become anxious than before.

In addition, in the first week after increasing my dose, around late afternoon or early evening, I would persistently feel light-headed and a little dizzy. I discussed this with my doctor and he said that this often happens when your calorie consumption drops significantly – your body isn't getting its usual fuel source, so it's confused, and the tank seems to be empty. Even after I got used to it, this feeling never entirely went away.

For between 5 and 10 per cent of people who take these drugs, the side effects are so extreme that they conclude it's not worth continuing. I spoke with a woman in Vermont named Sunny Naughton, who is four foot ten, and when she hit 190 pounds (13.6 stone), she realised her weight was spiralling out of control. So in 2018, she sought out – in desperation – Saxenda, an early GLP-1 agonist drug that had to be injected daily. In the first two months, she lost more than thirty pounds, but, she told me, 'I was sick all the time. Stomach cramps. Vomiting.' She found herself burping uncontrollably, with 'weird flavours', and 'there's a metallic taste in your mouth all the time'.

At work, she would end up rolling on the floor beneath her desk with stomach cramps so crippling that her colleague would have to drive her home. 'It just felt like someone was digging in and twisting your insides really tightly,' she said. It was so unlike anything she had experienced before that she felt 'an alien had gone into my stomach and was doing something in my body ... It felt like there was something living in my stomach that was tearing everything up and getting rid of whatever was in there, and then draining my body of energy.' For eight months, Sunny made herself endure it because the weight loss was so dramatic. But 'it was the worst physical illness that I ever felt ... From one to ten, it was fifty. It was just awful. And everyone around me was like, "Should you keep doing this?"' One day, she accidentally injected herself with a double dose. 'I was supposed to teach a class two days later, and I was so sick, I couldn't get out of bed. I was sweating. I was nauseous. I got myself into the bathtub. I was almost incoherent. I called my mother and said, "I might have to go to the ER." This medicine made me so sick.'

Not long afterwards, she told herself 'I need to live a natural life' and threw away her remaining pens. She rapidly put most of the weight back on, as does almost everyone who comes off these drugs, but the alien also seemed to leave her body.

Although my experience was far less severe, I wanted to understand why these side effects were happening. Carel Le Roux, one of the scientists who played a crucial role in developing these drugs, talked me through it. He likes to say that there are two kinds of drugs: drugs that don't work, and drugs that have side effects. You become constipated because the surge of GLP-1 slows down your gut and its emptying. The food and waste sit inside you for longer and find it harder to get out. Similarly, you burp because 'the valve that sits at the bottom of the stomach doesn't open as quickly. The air must go somewhere, so instead of it going down into the small intestine, people start burping.' You become nauseous because the drug creates a sensation of extreme satiety – that you are full and can't eat any more. The human brain struggles to distinguish between extreme satiety and sickness: the two signals get easily mixed up, which is why, even for people who aren't taking these drugs, after a really big meal you often feel a little nauseous.

But, he said, for the vast majority in the clinical trials, these side effects passed quite quickly. Their bodies got used to it and the negatives went away, or at least faded to a tolerable level. (At the moment, the drug companies are tweaking the drugs to reduce nausea, by adding a hormone named amylin. The clinical trials on that are taking place as I write this.)

Yet I didn't feel that my ambivalence could be fully explained by the side effects I was experiencing. Something more was going on, though it took me time to figure out what it was. Every time I upped my dose, the side effects got worse, but then they mostly eased off – so I felt confident that if I powered through them, they would, over time, diminish to little or nothing. So why didn't I feel as happy as I should? Why – in addition to moments of glee – did I feel moments of deep worry about what I was doing? Why was I looking a gift horse – effortless weight loss, the dream of humans down the ages – in the mouth?

I began to see the answer when I decided to go right back to where this story, for me, began. I asked: Why did I get fat in the first place? And more importantly, why did we – as a culture – get so much fatter, in a very short period of time?

I learned that we can't understand these drugs unless we first take a moment to understand the forces that made so many of us need them in the first place. It was only when I studied this question that some of the mysteries around these drugs began to be resolved.

2

Cheesecake Park
Why we gained weight

I was born in 1979, which is roughly the year that something unprecedented started to happen to human beings. For as long as our species has existed, there have always been some obese people. We know they were there because they crop up occasionally in the historical record – an ancient statue, a sixteenth-century painting, a Charles Dickens novel. They fell into a small number of categories. Some belonged to a tiny super-rich elite. For example, William the Conqueror, the English king in the eleventh century, gained so much weight that when he died and they tried to put his body into a stone tomb, his corpse exploded. Others almost certainly had extremely rare genetic conditions, which still exist. Some people cannot produce a hormone called leptin, and so they feel ravenously hungry all the time. Others have a condition called Prader-Willi syndrome, where they have some missing genetic material on a key chromosome, and almost literally can't stop eating. Wherever these obese people existed, they were regarded as very unusual, because they were so rare.

But according to scientists at the National Institutes of Health in the United States, this began to change in the late

1970s. Obesity had likely been rising very slowly since the turn of the twentieth century, but suddenly, it went supersonic. Between the year I was born and the year I turned twenty-one, obesity more than doubled in the United States, from 15 per cent to 30.9 per cent. The rate of severe obesity took a particularly disturbing turn: between my twenty-first birthday and my forty-first, it almost doubled. The average American adult weighs twenty-three pounds more than in 1960, and more than 70 per cent of all Americans are either overweight or obese. England has followed a similar trend. In 1980, 6 per cent of men were obese. By 2018, it was 27 per cent.

This is happening almost everywhere that experiences one crucial change, one I will come to in a moment. As a result, the World Health Organization says that obesity has nearly tripled globally since 1975. This has never happened before in the 300,000-year history of our species. It means we look different, move differently, and suffer from more and different illnesses. As Jerold Mande, the Harvard academic who designed the nutritional label displayed on all food in the US, told me: 'There was no genetic shift that happened in the 1970s or 80s. There was no massive change of willpower that occurred. Yet all of a sudden, people started gaining weight rapidly.' If you could build a time machine and bring our ancestors back from even the recent past to see us now, I think the thing that would shock them most is not our smartphones or fast cars but that we have been physically transformed. For a long time, whenever I piled on the pounds, I felt like I had personally failed – but it turned out I was in fact a wholly typical product of my times.

So I wanted to know: what happened to us? To solve any problem, it always helps to know how it was created. What spurred the need for Ozempic in the first place – and could it be fixed in other, less risky and expensive ways?

This change happened quickly enough to be shocking, but slowly enough that we seem to have accepted it without much fightback or friction. We slowly fattened together. If you blamed anyone, it was likely yourself: I'm not disciplined enough; I need more willpower. We tried a flurry of diets and exercise programmes. But mostly we uneasily accepted it, as if it was natural, or at least inevitable.

But there was at least one place where this change was vehemently contested – inside my own family. It was the source of extreme arguments, and a violent attempt to hold back the tide. The story of my childhood is weird in many ways, but I think it might serve as a microcosm to help us to see the forces that, in my fairly short lifetime, have changed us all.

~

My parents met when they were in their early twenties on the dance floor of a nightclub near Carnaby Street, in the West End of London, in 1967. They were both runaways.

My mother had grown up in the damp tenements of Scotland and she had been on course for the standard life it offered working-class women of her generation – marriage, semi-servitude, back-breaking work, all eased only by dry humour and lots of carbohydrates. One day her fiancé had abruptly broken off their engagement, and she decided it was the moment to make her lucky escape and flee to London.

My father had grown up in a wooden farmhouse on the side of a mountain in the Swiss Alps. His parents worked every waking hour farming their land and feeding their animals. All five of their children were expected, from the age of five, to toil on the farm too. My father believed there had to be more to life than feeding pigs, so he hitched his way across Europe, to where he heard there was a party happening in the British capital.

On the night they met, my father spoke around ten words of English, and my mother didn't speak a word of French or German. Even now, she will often cry and say: 'He seemed so nice when I couldn't understand what he was saying.' They had what my mother calls 'a series of one-night stands' – a concept I tried to explain to her does not make sense. She got pregnant, and they thought they had to get married. They had their first argument as a married couple as soon as she signed the marriage register. She used her maiden name. 'You idiot!' he shouted. 'That's not your name any more! Now you have my surname!' 'Fuck off!' she yelled back. They have been yelling at each other ever since. Once he learned English and she could understand what he was saying all the time, it got significantly worse.

My dad was a chef and together they travelled all over the world, where he would work in whatever kitchen would take him. He cooked in hotels in London, Berlin, Lausanne, Dallas, Alexandria, Tehran, Johannesburg and – in time for my birth – Glasgow. My dad was a chef at the Albany Hotel, and the very first photograph of me to appear in a newspaper is when I am around a year old, where he is wearing a chef's hat and spooning food into my mouth. In the picture, he is smiling. It is the first and last time I recall him smiling at anything I ate.

My parents came from diametrically opposed food cultures. In Kandersteg, the village in the Alps where my paternal ancestors have lived for centuries, you ate what you grew, what you fed, and what you killed. They planted and grew their own vegetables, and bred and slaughtered their own animals for meat. All food was freshly prepared from scratch on the day it was consumed. A researcher who compared food cultures across the world in the 1930s found that this was the healthiest one in the world, alongside the Aboriginal peoples of Australia.

In the Scottish working classes, food was totally different. My exhausted, beaten-down ancestors there were ahead of the global trend – they led the world in eating vast amounts of salted, fried carbohydrates. They wanted stodge, and lots of it. They needed food to be cheap, and they needed it to last a long time – so it was cooked in batches, and rarely eaten fresh. It's not a coincidence that this is the place that invented the concept of the deep-fried Mars bar and has been for many years one of the most obese nations in the developed world.

From the year of my birth on, the diet of the Western world suddenly shifted, from looking a lot like the one my father grew up with to closely resembling the one my mother grew up with. In the main, people stopped buying fresh ingredients and cooking them into meals. Instead, they started to buy food that was pre-packaged and pre-processed. That food was very different to what came before, in all sorts of crucial ways.

This change looked like a liberation to my mother and my maternal grandmother, who came to live with us because my mother was often seriously unwell. My grandmother had worked to the point of exhaustion since she was thirteen – cleaning toilets, scrubbing floors – and the arrival of the microwave was one of the happiest days of her life. 'It's food but *you don't have to do anything*!' she would say, clapping her hands with glee and waiting for that sweet, sweet ping. She and my mother fed me the products of this new industrialised food system, genuinely believing it was a bounteous gift both to them and to me. The tastes of those foods can make me moist-eyed with nostalgia even now: frozen Findus Crispy Pancakes, a kind of breaded envelope with pre-processed beef at its heart; Micro-Chips, a brand of fries that took only two minutes to heat up; Angel Delight, a pink powder you added to milk to make a sugary dessert.

My father was enraged and disgusted by this food. He would come home from a day's work cooking, and watch me eating a diet that to him didn't look like food at all. He would yell: 'He will die if he never eats vegetables!' My parents would scream at each other about it: she insisted that a child should enjoy food, while he insisted that enjoyment had nothing to do with it and that the child was being poisoned. He had no way to communicate his concern in a way that I, as a kid, could understand as anything other than humiliation. He had been raised in a Swiss environment where you didn't try to persuade children of anything – you threatened them, you frightened them, and if necessary, you physically forced them. On Swiss farms, kids were deliberately hardened through brutality: for example, when my dad was a child and his cat had kittens, he was made to watch as his father drowned them all in a bucket one by one. In our house, he would cook fresh food and when I refused it and asked for more Angel Delight, he would pin me down and physically try to force my mouth open so he could shove salad leaves in.

This is how his own harsh childhood had prepared him to treat kids – but it clashed with the world I was living in.

Everyone else I knew was eating what I ate – why was he objecting? Every time I switched on the TV, there were ads telling me that this food was fantastic – what was wrong with him? Every time I went to school, the lunches were equally fatty and carby and fried – would they feed it to us if it was so bad? I could only experience his fresh food as an inexplicable assault.

By this time, we were living in the suburbs of north London, and we started to be encircled for the first time by fast-food outlets. They were opening everywhere – a McDonald's, a KFC, a Wimpy bar. The Chicken McNugget was invented when I was two years old. I found that I could torment my father by refusing to eat any evening meal unless he drove me to KFC or McDonald's and got me some of this food. It became a tug of wills between us. Sometimes, he would capitulate, and watch me gnawing through fried drumsticks and ask, 'What is wrong with you?' Other times, he would win, and I would go hungry, until my grandmother secretly snuck me some microwaved food late at night, whispering: 'Don't tell him.'

Nothing about the new style of eating made sense to my father. When he was a child, nobody ate snacks. I expected a snack every few hours. He had grown up knowing where almost all his food came from, and he was puzzled that I had no more curiosity about it than where my electricity or clothes came from. Back in Kandersteg, it was regarded as greedy to eat more than a small portion even at mealtimes. In this new food culture, you could stuff your face forever. My father was appalled at how fast I ate my food, screaming at me to slow down. To my mother and grandmother, who had grown up in poverty, the way I ate made sense. Why wouldn't you take food while you can? Who turns down a meal? Who wants to make preparing food more onerous than it has to be?

Every day, my father felt like he had been catapulted without his consent out of a healthy food culture into a sick one and it infuriated him. To me, it felt like I had a Flintstones father in a Jetsons age, trying to drag me back to eating raw dinosaur meat. One time, he brought home a pig's snout, and tried to force me and my sister to eat it, as we screamed and cried.

Since he was out working almost all the time, I would cram my preferred food into my mouth without restraint – a mixture of Cheesy Wotsits, salt and vinegar chipsticks, Coco Pops, Rice Krispies, snowballs (marshmallow surrounded by chocolate), mini rolls. In a very stressful environment – with my mother unwell, my father full of scorn, and both of them often enraged – I got great comfort from this food, and I had no sense that I should restrain my consumption of it.

I took pleasure primarily in one particular physical sensation: stuffing myself. Stuffing is a very particular form of eating – it is when you eat to the point that you are full, and then deliberately keep eating more and more and more. As I did this, I would feel it stretching me inside, pushing outwards on my stomach and upwards on my oesophagus. These sensations soothed me. Stuffing is the opposite of savouring: you pay no attention to the food or its flavour, you just pile it in. I only occasionally got a sense that this was not how everyone ate. One time, a boy at my school with a touch of entrepreneurial zeal started to bring in cakes and sell slices of them at break time. I bought slice after slice, and I remember him telling me to slow down because I would make myself sick, and I wondered what he meant. After school, I would go to McDonald's every day on the way home, and gorge myself. Then my grandmother and I would lie on our sofa, watching Australian soap operas and inhaling snacks.

There were times when my mother and grandmother were away and I was left alone with my dad, and all he would prepare was the fresh food he thought I should eat. I refused to eat any of it. I would rather starve.

I had absolute confidence that I was attuned to the culture I lived in, and my father was outside it. After the collapse of the Soviet Union, its last leader, Mikhail Gorbachev, appeared in an ad for Pizza Hut. He had gone from ruling a Communist empire that covered a quarter of the earth's surface to promoting greasy slices of processed cheese. It was, I thought proudly, a symbol of the victory of our way of life.

Strangely enough, none of this eating made me fat, not until my late teens. I had a round face and chubby cheeks but that was all. I never thought about any of this having any relevance to my health. Indeed, if you had asked me, I would have said I took unusually good care of my health – I drank Diet Coke, not the full-sugar version, and with my mother, every morning, I would swallow a fistful of multivitamins, which I somehow believed magically cancelled out everything else.

Perhaps this sounds like an extreme story to you, and in some ways it is – but my family's experience is only really unusual in two ways. Firstly, I leaned harder and faster into the new culture of processed junk food than other people, and secondly, there was an adult present who tried, in his own deeply flawed way, to stop it and drag me back to the food culture that almost all other humans had experienced for our 300,000 years on earth.

~

Because I was born into this revolution in how humans eat, it was hard for me to see how drastic this change was, and how different the food I ate was to that consumed by my father, and grandparents, and ancestors. My father kept asking me: Where do you think this shitty food comes from?

It turns out the answer to my dad's question is key to understanding how this food affects us. When he posed it to me, I didn't care, but if I had thought about it, I suspect a mental picture would have come easily. Obviously, somewhere there was essentially a big, busy kitchen, where they made this stuff, and then shipped it to our local supermarket. The gap between 'home-cooked' and 'factory-prepared' was, surely, only one of scale. He made stuff in a small kitchen. I ate food made in a big kitchen. The end. But a decade ago, the journalist Joanna Blythman managed to get into several of the food factories that have cropped up across the Western world, in anonymous industrial parks on the edges of our cities, to see how what we eat is actually made. In her excellent book *Swallow This*, she describes what she found – and shows how wrong my assumption was.

Once inside, she discovered that the places where our food is produced look nothing like a kitchen. They reminded her of a car plant, an oil refinery, or the missile-launching pad at the end of a James Bond film. Vast amounts of unrecognisable chemicals are pumped through processors and into vats through metallic tubes. The people in charge of these factories don't use the word 'cooking' at all; they refer to what they do as 'manufacturing' food, and that is how it looked to Joanna.

Everything is stripped down to its component parts (or a replica of them), and then assembled into food. Almost nothing is what you expect it to be. If you watched the making of, say, a strawberry milkshake, you would expect at some point to see, somewhere, a strawberry, being pulped and processed. But in fact, in a typical strawberry-flavoured milkshake, the flavouring alone is made up of fifty chemicals – none of which is a strawberry.

The manufacturers are doing this for one reason above all others. Fresh food rots quickly, and these factories are preparing food that needs to be able to sit on a supermarket shelf for weeks, months or years. To achieve this, they have to dramatically alter it. If you pump food full of sugar and fat, it reduces bacterial growth, and if you add salt, it lasts longer on the shelf without rotting. So our food is filled with unheard-of amounts of all three.

Then there is a further challenge. To make food cheaply at this scale, you have to strip it down to its chemical elements, get them delivered in bulk, and assemble them to make an approximation of the food that we expect – a kind of ersatz curry, a replica of a cheese and tomato pizza, made out of dozens or hundreds of chemicals. But this process creates food, Joanna explains, that doesn't quite look or taste like food at first: 'The hard fact of the matter is that the extreme temperatures and stress involved in industrial food manufacture do grievous bodily harm to natural ingredients, irrevocably damaging their intrinsic textures, flavours and aromas.' They appear dull and inedible. So it is necessary to add large numbers of colourings to make them look like the original form of the food. For example, 'a dash of red makes pasta sauce look as if it contains more tomato than it really does'. These industrial processes often leave the food tasting metallic or bitter, so they then need to be pumped full of '6,000 food additives – flavourings, glazing agents, improvers, anti-caking agents, solvents, preservatives, colourings, acids, emulsifiers, releasing agents, antioxidants, thickeners, bleaching agents, sweeteners, chelators'. As one food scientist put it, 'Our job is to make something taste like something, even if it is not.'

One of the most commonly used artificial flavourings in our food is vanillin, a fake form of vanilla chemically constructed out of petrochemicals, wood pulp or sawdust. Food with a buttery taste gets there not with butter but with a 0.02 per cent 'butter extract', buffeted by large numbers of additives. Walking around the places that put all this together, Joanna was struck that 'it is actually relatively rare to see anything that looks much like food as we know it'.

After she had spent time in these food construction sites, she managed to get herself smuggled into one of the big food industry trade shows that are closed to outsiders. It was an event named Food Ingredients, where the corporations that own these factories source their raw materials. One typical stand explained that the chemical components they were selling for inclusion in human food had many other uses: they boasted that their chemicals could be used in bakery products and meat, but also in 'fly spray, air freshener, shower sealant, deodorant, computer casing, scratch-resistant car coating, paint and glue'. Joanna learned that to make meat last on supermarket shelves, it has to be pumped full of water – but the water only stays in if you combine it with 'meat glue', a substance as gross as it sounds. Some other meat is heavily injected with ammonia hydroxide gas to kill the bacteria that have built up, creating something a food executive called 'pink slime', which makes up 15 per cent of some minced beef items. A similar product named 'meat slurry' – made of liquefied chicken and emulsifier – is used to make the cheapest chicken nuggets.

The products that emerge from this manufacturing process have sometimes been named 'Frankenfood', or 'food-like substances' as the writer Michael Pollan calls them. Joanna writes: 'The resulting pizza, curry and cheesecake retain only a blurry, faint memory of the freshly prepared equivalent. These pre-processed labour saving ingredients are simply not fresh, and storage has robbed them of their initial sparkle.'

But the additives that are pumped into them create a new kind of deliciousness, one that my palate was trained to crave. The scientists working for these food manufacturers have carefully studied how to create what they call 'bliss-points' – moments in the consumption of these foods when we will feel a sugar-kick, or a moment of mouth-bliss, or a wildly exciting aftertaste, all constructed by their shower of chemicals. They've spent years finding the perfect combination of crunchiness and cream, of sugar and chocolate, of something popping on your tongue.

As I interviewed people who have studied how industrially processed food is made and is now affecting us, I felt lost. They were telling me that, all my life, I had been eating an unnatural chemical stew, dripping with stuff that is unseen in nature and was unknown to my ancestors.

It meant that the food I grew up loving was, in some strange sense, not really food at all.

I felt unmoored, and disorientated – like I was discovering that my oldest and most beloved friends had secretly been brutal criminals all along.

~

Many of the scientists who have studied this food say that this new kind of industrially assembled form affects us very differently from the old type of food. There is one effect I learned about, more than any other, that I kept reflecting on in relation to Ozempic and the other weight-loss drugs. To understand it, I think it helps to look at one experiment in particular.

In the year 2000, a young scientist named Paul Kenny moved from Dublin to San Diego to continue his neuroscientific research. He noticed something pretty quickly. In the main, Americans don't eat like Irish people. They eat more, and they consume more sugars and fats in particular. Paul was thrown at first, but he soon assimilated – and within two years, he had gained thirty pounds. 'I was like – oh my lord, what is going on?' he told me.

He rose to become the chair of the Department of Neuroscience at the Icahn School of Medicine at Mount Sinai in New York, and on the way, he grew curious about something. Did this different American diet change your brain? Once you start to eat in this way – lots of processed, fatty, sugary foods – might it be harder to stop? With his colleagues, he designed an experiment to test this.

They raised a group of lab rats, and fed them nothing but pre-prepared rat chow. 'It's healthy. It's balanced,' Paul said – the lab rat equivalent of what my father grew up eating. When this was all they had, the rats would eat until they were full, and then their natural instincts would kick in, and they would stop. They never became obese.

Then he introduced the rats to the hyper-American diet. He bought some cheesecake and Snickers bars, and fried up some bacon. He split the rats into two groups. The first group was given access to the junkiest American food for one hour a day. The second group was given access to it almost all day. Both groups also, at the same time, had access to as much of the healthy rat chow as they wanted.

You might call these cages Cheesecake Park – a place where the rats got to eat just like us. Paul watched as the rats sniffed the cheesecake and the Snickers and the bacon, and they began to eat. And eat. And eat.

The rats who only had an hour with the cheesecake would 'dip their head into it' the moment it arrived 'and munch all the way through' until it was totally gone, Paul said. 'The head would be slick with cheesecake. They'd gorge themselves,' and emerge 'smothered in cheesecake'. The rats who had access to it all the time would eat even more, and they consumed it differently. They would eat some, leave it for a little while, then come back and eat some more. They were frequently topping up with sugar and fat.

For both groups, as soon as they had the American diet, they lost interest in the healthy old rat chow. They shunned it. It bored them. The rats who got cheesecake for an hour a day would get just a third of their calories from the rat chow. The rats who had cheesecake all the time got just 5 per cent of their calories from ordinary rat chow. They lost their ability to control their eating. Their old instincts, which kept them healthy, stopped working. They simply gorged.

As a result, 'they really gained a lot of weight, very quickly', Paul said. Within six weeks, their obesity rates skyrocketed, and they started to have health problems. 'They're hyperleptinaemic. They're hyperglycaemic. They have all these markers for obesity.' He was struck by how quickly they flipped for the new food. 'They really chow down very, very quickly, and they look markedly different ... Within a few days, they are different animals. Their physiology is profoundly altered, very, very quickly. That was really quite striking. And shocking.' Out of all the unhealthy food options, they went especially mad for the cheesecake. 'What is it about this food?' Paul asked. 'It was the most energy-dense food we could find that wasn't actually pure oil. It was basically emulsified oil that was kept together with sugar. This blend of fat and sugar was just amazing. The ultimate food, if you will.'

Then, once the rats were extremely fat and had got used to eating the processed food for a few months, Paul did something harsh. He took it all away. He abruptly cut off the supply of junk food, and the rats were left with just the nutritious, healthy rat chow they had been consuming all their lives until recently.

Paul was fairly confident about what would happen next. They would eat larger portions of the standard rat chow than before, proving that the junk food had expanded their appetites and made them crave more. This would be a worrying effect, to be sure.

But that's not what happened. What actually took place was more extreme. In the absence of their beloved junk food, the rats refused to eat almost anything. To Paul, they seemed lost and angry. 'They basically starved rather than eat this other food. They rejected it. They thought it was horrendous.'

It was like they had forgotten what real food was, and no longer recognised it as food at all. 'You begin to see this dramatic weight loss. The animals are really starving themselves,' he explained. It was only when they reached the point where if 'they didn't eat it, they'd starve to death, [and] they had no choice' that they returned reluctantly to the nutritious food, eating a little of the old rat chow.

So before they were exposed to the new American diet, they had an ability to naturally limit how much they ate, and even though they had an abundance of food, they never became obese. But once they were exposed to it – high sugar and fat, all in a highly processed package – the rats became obsessed, ate far more than they had before, gained a huge amount of weight, and got sick. And after trying it, they had to be starving before they would go back to the way they used to eat.

As he told me this, I thought about when my mother and grandmother were away, and my dad prepared salads for me, and I cried and went to my room hungry.

~

Paul then discovered something else this food did to the rats.

He ran the experiment again, and this time with a twist. He set up two cages: one where the rats got standard chow and the other where the rats got cheesecake. Then he rigged up the floor of both cages, and set a trap. Occasionally, while eating, the rats would get a nasty electric shock. At the same time, they would be shown a yellow light. You don't have to do this for long before the rats start to associate seeing a yellow light with being electrocuted, and they become very frightened of it.

Then, one day, Paul gave them their food – rat chow for one group, cheesecake for the other – and showed them the yellow light, but didn't electrocute them. He was making them very afraid, without triggering the physical effects of the electrocution, to see what would happen. The rats who had only been given rat chow freaked out and ran away. The pleasure of the food was beaten by a desire to avoid the pain of the electric shock. But the rats who had been given cheesecake stayed and carried on eating. They were 'ignoring the warning they had been trained to fear', as Paul put it. The rats wanted their hit of sugar and fat, and the fear of a painful electric shock didn't deter them. If you are exposed to this food for a while, Paul concluded, the desire for it is so great that you will ignore all sorts of negative consequences.

~

Experiments like this have been conducted many times with rats, and scientists keep finding similar outcomes. For example, rats normally hate stepping out into the open, and will always try to stay close to boundaries or walls. But if you feed them Fruit Loops, afterwards, whenever they see them, they want them so badly they will walk into the open to consume them. To give another example, Barry Levin, a professor at the New Jersey Medical School, bred a strain of rats whose genes predisposed them to resisting obesity – rats who were, in our terms, naturally skinny. Once they were unleashed on a high-fat, high-sugar diet, they became just as obese as the other rats.

~

Once the experiment was over, Paul could never bring himself to eat cheesecake again. 'Not,' he said with a shake of the head, 'after seeing rats gorge on it.'

~

After years of raging at the way I ate, my father slowly gave in to it. He quit his job as a cook, and became a bus driver. He started to eat worse food, gained a lot of weight, and had to have heart surgery in his early seventies.

I pictured him on his hospital bed, wired with tubes, and thought: It's very hard to resist Cheesecake Park.

3

The Death and Rebirth of Satiety

The strange connection between processed food and the new drugs

It is clear that this new kind of factory-assembled, ultra-processed food is triggering a frenzy in many of us that is like the one those rats experienced. Dunkin' Donuts now sells enough doughnuts every day to circle the earth twice, and twenty years ago, Ronald McDonald was the second most recognised figure for American kids, beaten only by Santa Claus. More people recognise the Golden M as the symbol for McDonald's than the number of people who recognise the cross as a symbol of Christianity. On the Las Vegas Strip, there is a giant replica of the Statue of Liberty, but at its base it does not say 'Give us your poor, your huddled masses, yearning to breathe free'. Instead, there are people handing out vouchers for discounted meals at Denny's. Every time I walk past it, I think – yes, that's the true symbol of our culture in the twenty-first century. You're not here to be free; you're here to eat.

The Harvard adjunct professor of nutrition Jerold Mande told me: 'There's something about the food we're eating, and the redesign of the food, that's telling us to keep eating, even though your body should have told you to stop.' This effect is at the core of why so many of us now feel we need weight-loss drugs.

But why does this food unhinge our appetites? The first glimmer of an answer was discovered in 1995, when the Australian researcher and doctor Susanna Holt, working at the University of Sydney, decided to figure out: which foods make you feel full, and which ones leave you wanting more? She gave people a 240-calorie portion of thirty-eight different foods, and tracked both how full it made them feel, and how long it took them to get that feeling of fullness. She found one type of food makes you feel full very fast: whole foods, the kind my dad grew up eating – things like steak, potatoes, fresh fruit, fish. You eat them, you have enough, and you want to stop. At the other end of the spectrum, she found that a different kind of food really doesn't make you feel full for long: most processed foods, the kind I grew up eating – biscuits, boxed cereals, cakes, flavoured yogurts, croissants. You eat them and you want more and more and more.

The foods that used to dominate our diets made us feel full, while the foods that now dominate our diets leave us feeling there's a hole in our stomachs. Paul Kenny, who carried out the Cheesecake Park experiment, told me that when confronted with this kind of food 'it is hard for our bodies to really provide the feedback to us where you have that feeling of being full and sated'.

~

This was a really important concept, one I heard from almost everyone I interviewed about the shift in our diets. Satiety, or the feeling of no longer wanting more, is not a word we use much in everyday life, but I kept hearing it in two contexts. The first was the science of factory-assembled food – because this food, it turns out, is designed to undermine satiety. The second was in the science of the new weight-loss drugs – because they are designed to boost satiety. I only slowly began to trace the connections between them.

~

When you don't feel sated, you eat more, and over time, gain weight. By reading through the scientific research and interviewing the experts, I learned that there are, in fact, seven ways in which this new kind of processed food could be undermining our sense of satiety. One of the people who helped me to understand this is Tim Spector, professor of genetic epidemiology at King's College London. He uncovered these insights in part by studying thousands of pairs of identical twins, trying to discover why some of them gained weight when others didn't. If you could figure this out, he reasoned, you might be able to figure out why this is happening to so many of us. I interviewed him in his office, where dozens of photographs of identical twins stared down at me, smiling. The effect was slightly eerie. As I avoided their gaze, Tim helped me to see some of the reasons I have been so damn hungry all my life – far more than my father, or grandfather, or great-grandfather.

The first way that ultra-processed food undermines our satiety is strangely simple. You chew it less. It is, Tim explained, 'generally very soft … It is adult baby food.' When you eat, your body gradually registers that food is coming in and sends you the signal that you've had enough. If you have to chew your food and it takes longer to eat it, the signal to stop kicks in at the right time, when you are sated. But when you don't have to chew – when it all just slips down your gullet with disarming ease – you don't get the signal to stop until you've gone too far and gorged yourself. Chewing, Tim said, is a necessary brake on overeating, and processed food has tampered with the brakes.

As he said this, I thought of something. For my books, I often take long road trips around the US, and a few years ago I became obsessed with a product sold in most 7-Elevens called Fruit Squeeze. It's a soft green metallic pack that's filled with around half a dozen pulped apples that you spray directly into your mouth. When I have to eat a whole apple, bite by bite, and chew it into a pulp for myself, I never eat more than two in a row. But with these squirty tubes of semi-liquified apples, I can spray dozens of apples into my mouth in a row, as if I've just won the Formula One and it's champagne. Thanks to food processing, most of our food is now less like an apple and more like that Fruit Squeeze.

The second way our satiety is being undermined is that these manufactured foods often contain that uniquely powerful combination of sugar, fat and carbs – and this seems to activate something primal in us. We go crazy for it, in a way we don't for other kinds of food. Dr Giles Yeo, an obesity researcher who I interviewed in his lab at the University of Cambridge, told me his hunch about why that is. There is, so far as he is aware, likely only one foodstuff available in abundance in nature 'where you have carbs and fat naturally mixed together as a unit' – and it's breast milk. This is the first food almost all of us consume. It soothes us. As a species, humans didn't access this seemingly unique sugar–fat combo after we've been weaned – until now. So we lap at it like an infant at the breast, and gorge.

The third way is that processed food seems to affect your energy levels differently. When you consume food, your body breaks it down into blood sugar – your body's main source of energy – and sends it all over your body to power you through the day. When your blood sugar levels dip, you run out of energy and get the signal that you want to eat again. The kind of food my dad grew up eating releases energy slowly and steadily into your body, and if you eat it, your blood sugar will dip two or three times a day, around mealtimes, and you'll be hungry only then. But if you eat the kind of food I grew up eating, something very different happens. Most of us have had the experience where you inhale a box of Pringles and feel full – for about half an hour, and then you're ravenous for more. That is because Pringles give you a sudden shot of energy and blood sugar – and then your blood sugar crashes quickly, and you're hungry again in a flash. Tim explained that 'if you're having lots of short peaks' like this, 'you're much more likely to trigger appetite', over and over again. As so much of our diet has come to resemble Pringles, we end up living on what the nutritionist Dale Pinnock calls a roller coaster of energy spikes and energy crashes throughout the day, triggering much more hunger.

The fourth way is that processed food lacks two things we really need – protein and fibre. The effect this is having has been investigated by David Raubenheimer, a professor of nutritional ecology at the University of Sydney. Protein is a complex molecule that we all need to build muscles and healthy bones, and David wondered if there was a deep underlying reason why eating low-protein processed foods – as most of us do these days – could drive us to overeat. What if we have more than one kind of hunger? We all know we have a natural hunger for calories to give us energy, but the body also knows that for it to function properly it also needs protein. So he asked – what if your body makes you hungry not just for calories in general, but also for protein, and it leaves you feeling unsatisfied until you get enough of both? If this was true, it could cause a problem in an environment full of processed foods. Imagine a table where, to the left, you have the kind of high-protein meals my dad grew up eating, and to the right, you have the low-protein meals I grew up eating. To get the same amount of protein into your system, the meal to the right would have to be much bigger. You would have to eat much more.

To figure out if this was true, David designed a small but clever experiment. He split people into two groups, and one was given a high-protein diet, and the other was given a low-protein diet. Both were told they could eat as much as they wanted. They were then monitored, to see how much they consumed. It turned out that both groups ate the same amount of protein – but to get it, the people eating the processed food had to consume 35 per cent more calories in total. This, he told me, was proof that when we consume processed foods, we eat more of them 'to get our fill of protein'.

At the same time, fibre is a type of carbohydrate that we can't fully digest, so when you eat it, it takes longer for food to pass through your body, and your whole digestive process is slowed down. David explained to me that (like chewing) this acts as 'a brake' on eating. When you don't have much fibre in your diet, you'll get hungry again more quickly, and eat more. Processed foods are generally low in fibre.

The fifth way is that a lot of the drinks we now consume contain chemicals that may be actively triggering us to be more hungry. I only really began to understand this when I studied the science of sodas. In my lifetime, the consumption of fizzy drinks has roughly tripled. It's much easier to consume lots of calories in liquid form than from solid food: think about how easily you could consume a 2,000-calorie sugary drink, compared to the same amount of calories in the form of a large steak and fries. This surge of sodas has caused a tsunami of increased calorie consumption – for every extra soft drink a child consumes a day, there is a 60 per cent boost to the risk of them becoming obese.

But I was quite smug about this. I thought that out of all the causes of obesity, this was one where I had wisely dodged a bullet. As I mentioned earlier, I don't drink sugary sodas. I drink the diet kind, all stamped with 'zero calories' on the can. I was pure.

Yet here's the strange thing. The science is mixed and not always of the highest quality, but some rigorous studies seem to suggest that even these diet drinks can cause you to gain a significant amount of weight. For example, Susan Swithers, professor of psychological sciences at Purdue University in Indiana, has carried out experiments where she gives rats either sugar or artificial sweeteners – and the rats given artificial sweeteners gained *more* weight. She said the sweeteners seem to cause 'metabolic derangement' in rats. When I first read this, I thought it couldn't be true. How could a zero-calorie drink make you fatter than a sugary one that's crammed with calories?

Tim investigated this – and he started by experimenting on himself. He wired himself up with a glucose monitor, and drank a mixture of water and one of the most common artificial sweeteners. These chemicals are marketed as 'inert' – that is, they don't have any effect on your body, and are just passing through, like good tourists who leave the countryside in the same pristine condition as when they arrived. But as Tim watched his glucose levels, he was startled. They surged by more than 30 per cent. He told me: 'It's obviously not inert. It's doing something.' In a study published in 2022, a team of Israeli scientists split 120 people into groups. Twice a day for two weeks, they gave them either one of four artificial sweeteners or real sugar. The artificial sweeteners had a striking effect. Two of them raised blood sugar for everyone who drank them, and all four of them altered the bacteria in the people's guts in the way that happens when you have high blood sugar.

What causes this? It is in part, Tim suspects, because these chemicals have an effect on your brain. You drink something sweet, and it expects a surge of energy from sugar. Everything in our evolution primes you for it. When it doesn't come – when your brain realises it's been tricked – it responds by making you more hungry, to give it that fresh surge of energy it was expecting, and so 'you suddenly want cake'. Susan's groundbreaking studies have led her to believe that the presence of artificial sweeteners in our diets might be one of the big drivers of the obesity crisis.

The sixth factor is one that took me a while to really understand. This new kind of food has done something unprecedented: it has separated flavour from the underlying quality of our food. The nutritionist Jerold Mande explained this to me patiently. Over hundreds of thousands of years, he said, we evolved to have something called 'nutritional wisdom'. When our ancestors encountered something potentially edible in the past, they had a well-honed set of instincts to help them decide: do I eat this, or not? If it's sweet and soft, for example, it's likely fresh fruit, which is good for me, so I should eat it. 'We have millions of receptors in our nose and our mouth, essentially like a barcode reader,' Jerold said. 'It allows us, every time we eat something, to know what's in this food we're eating. It allows us to be nutritionally wise. It allows us to know that if we're not getting enough vitamin C or vitamin D, it'll lead us to that, and we'll eat it.' But the new form of food, he said, has scrambled all that. Food constructed in factories has 'separated the flavours from the foods. So the flavours tell you nothing.' Now the sweetness doesn't indicate fresh fruit. It can indicate a marshmallow, or a microwave lasagne, or a 3,000-calorie banana milkshake. Indeed, the system that used to tell you to eat fruit now tells you to eat Fruit Loops.

This means that our instincts – which guided us so wisely for so long – are now like a fritzing GPS that used to tell you how to drive home but is now telling you to drive off a cliff. What used to guide us to safety – and still would, in an environment filled with natural foods – instead pulls us towards sickness.

The seventh factor is that these foods seem to cause your gut to malfunction, in ways that undermine satiety. Tim has been at the forefront of studying this, and he explained that at the bottom of your intestines, there is a part of your body that is just as important as your brain. It is your gut microbiome. This 'is where most of your gut microbes live. They're sitting there, in the dark, in your colon, and there are hundreds of trillions of them.' They break down the food you eat, and release into your body all sorts of chemicals that are essential for you to live and function fully. They are 'absolutely crucial for your immune system, for fighting ageing, for your metabolism, for your energy control, and digesting food and getting the right things from it. You can't live without it. The healthier it is, the healthier you are.' Its health, crucially, comes from its diversity – the broader the range of healthy bugs living in your gut, the better it works.

But something very strange has happened to our guts. We now have vastly less diverse gut microbiomes than our ancestors. In fact, the average person has 'lost about 40 per cent' of the diverse life in our microbiomes, Tim said. Why would this be? To fully operate, your gut needs to be fed with a big, diverse array of types of food – ideally, roughly thirty different types of plant a week. But processed and junk food is made out of a few very limited building blocks: 'Eighty per cent of processed food is made up of just four ingredients – corn, wheat, soy and meat,' he explains. His research has shown that if you start to eat processed food, then within a few days, the health of your gut starts to dramatically change.

Starved of diversity, our guts sicken, like a garden sprayed with a pesticide. After leading research on this for decades, Tim has come to believe we are 'poisoning' our microbes with 'junk food, sweeteners and sugar'. As a result, our guts are malfunctioning, and are not able to control our appetite or energy as well as they did in the past. This, he believes, is 'likely to be responsible for much of our obesity epidemic'.

~

All this combines to have a shocking effect: one study found that processed foods make you eat, on average, 500 calories more every day than if you eat only similar non-processed foods. That's roughly the equivalent of adding a whole Big Mac to your daily diet. Now imagine that stretched over your whole life. Except I didn't have to imagine it. I felt bewildered as I realised these factors had been affecting me since I was a toddler. We eat, at least in part, to dial down our hunger. But I now saw that, all these years, I had been eating in a way that dialled *up* my hunger. It was like I had been trying to deal with my thirst by drinking seawater.

I started to think about this in relation to something else that has been taking place while we got fatter. Over the past fifty years, the agricultural industry has become really good at making many of the animals they own as big and bulky as possible. They do this for a few reasons. The bigger an animal gets, the more meat they have on their bones – you can carve more products out of a fat cow than a leaner one. At the same time, one of the biggest costs for this industry is housing the animals. The sooner you can get them to the weight you want, the lower those costs will be. The industry has been unbelievably efficient at achieving this mass fattening. Thirty years ago, it took twelve weeks for a factory-farmed chicken to reach its slaughter weight, but now it only takes five to six weeks. Broiler chickens are three times higher in fat today than they were when I was born, and the standard factory-farmed turkey now has such an obese chest that it can barely stand up.

So how did they do it? It turns out it was partly by restricting the animals' movement – lots of them can't even turn round in their cages. But even more importantly, they totally transformed their diets. If you feed a cow the wholefood it evolved to eat – grass – it will take a year longer to reach its slaughter weight than if you feed it something different: a newly invented kind of ultra-processed feed, made up of grains, chemicals, hormones and antibiotics. Because the animals don't like the taste of this fake food, the agricultural corporations often add artificial sweetness to it – Jell-O powder is popular, especially with a strawberry-banana flavouring. When you mix a sweet-tasting formula like this into their processed food, lambs will rapidly add 30 per cent to their body weight.

If you deliberately want to make an animal fat, you take away what its ancestors ate, and give it an ultra-processed and artificially sweetened replica instead. In other words – Big Agriculture does to animals precisely what the processed food industry is doing to us and our children every day.

~

As I walked out of Tim Spector's office and saw all those twins staring down at me one last time, I thought about his warning that as a result of so many of these factors, we are now living in a 'perfect obesity storm'. If ultra-processed food was a drug, he said, it would be taken off the market, because it would be regarded as too dangerous for people to use.

~

In the first few months of my research for this book, I interviewed people about what I thought of as two quite different topics. I talked to scientists who investigate how our food affects us, and I spoke with scientists about how the new generation of weight-loss drugs affects us. I thought of these as parallel tracks. But the same word kept cropping up at every step of the way, the one mentioned earlier: satiety. They started to seem less like separate tracks, and more like braided plaits.

Carel Le Roux, one of the scientists who developed these drugs, told me that people in the field often call GLP-1 and the other gut-chemicals 'satiety hormones', because this is precisely the sensation they seem to restore to people. Daniel Drucker, who played a key role in discovering GLP-1, told me that many people had 'given up ever having that feeling of satiety again' – until the drugs switched them back on.

The connections began to seem obvious. We have for forty years been consuming food that systematically undermines our satiety. Now, in response, we are demanding to be given drugs that give us back that lost sense of satiety. One produced the other. If this transformation in our food supply had not happened, the market for weight-loss drugs would be confined to a tiny number of people.

Once I realised this, my decision to start taking Ozempic began to seem ridiculous to me. Michael Lowe is a professor of clinical psychology at Drexel University in Philadelphia, and he has been one of the world's leading researchers into hunger for forty years. He is an animated man in his seventies who can look back on a lifetime of studying diet from every angle, and as we spoke, he helped me to connect the dots. These weight-loss drugs, he said, are 'an artificial solution to an artificial problem ... Obesity is an artificial problem in the sense that [we now eat] highly energy-dense foods that normally [don't exist] in nature. There was virtually none in our hunter-gatherer days. And now we've come up with an artificial solution, which is to fix the artificially undermined satiety through an artificially designed drug.'

Something is wrong, he believes, 'any time a society has a problem that everyone acknowledges is heavily based on the environment, and turns increasingly to treating it in a medical way'. It leads us to neglect what is causing the problem in the first place. 'If you find yourself in a ditch, the first thing you want to do is stop digging. We're still digging.' All the food companies are still finding ways to stuff us with even more irresistible foods. 'The pills, of course, are doing nothing about the environment.' The food industry finds ways to make our kids as fat as possible as young as possible, and then we scramble years later to fix the problem not in the society but inside our own guts.

The answer to a problem caused by a toxic food system is, Michael believes, to fix the food system. This is extremely hard to do as an isolated individual, but as a society, if we are determined, we can do it. (I later learned there are places that have actually done this, as you'll see.) It is possible, he insists, but 'basically, Western governments have mostly given up. That's what concerns me. We live in a world of medical marvels, curing us of all kinds of diseases. But where do you draw the line to say "let's live however we want, and we'll just depend on the pharmaceutical industry to save us from ourselves"? That's also what we're doing … As a culture, I'm afraid we have given up on the whole idea of prevention.' Instead, we choose risky quick fixes.

'Part of me says be careful what you wish for. Is this going to be our approach to "coping" with the obesity epidemic? We're going to design more and more expensive [and] permanent treatments?'

He sighed. 'Maybe I'm just out of touch. Maybe I'm using the values that I grew up with. But we're not supposed to just willingly go into a future where we don't even try to change ourselves – meaning our society, our restaurants, our food companies, our children. We don't even try.' Instead of trying to solve the problem we just drug ourselves. 'Is that how you want to advance as a species?' When he looks at these drugs, he thinks, 'It's like a child's answer to life's problems. You don't change what's producing it . . . It's like a magical kingdom where you wish it, and it comes true.' The alternative is to actually solve the underlying problem, 'so that fifty years from now, 80 per cent of us aren't on weight-loss drugs'.

I felt like he had articulated my latent fears really well. Many other people who have studied obesity for a long time have been issuing similar warnings. Robert Lustig, a professor of paediatrics who for decades has been at the forefront of warning that our food is killing us, told the *Guardian* he believes these drugs are 'a Band-Aid. Giving a medicine just to do weight loss is basically closing your eyes and hoping for the best.' The answer, he insisted, is to change the food supply. Henry Dimbleby, who led the British government's inquiry into how to solve the obesity crisis, warned that the country cannot 'drug its way out of the problem'. He argued that relying on this approach was 'reckless', and said that instead it should follow the lead of Japan, which has kept obesity down in a very different way – one that I would soon see for myself.

I believe in facing difficult problems without flinching and then tackling them at their root. I had written books before about why we should reject superficial solutions to our crises of depression, anxiety and addiction, and focus primarily on dealing with their underlying psychological and social causes. I was starting to feel that taking Ozempic was a betrayal of my values.

Every time I injected myself, I felt fraudulent.

But then something happened that made me think again.

~

Seven years ago, one of my closest friends – I'll call her Judy – got breast cancer, and nearly died. I was there with her through the bouts of chemo, her hair loss, her double mastectomy, and then (thank God) her full recovery. Since I helped her through her health crisis, she has, in a loving way, been telling me that she is worried about my own health. 'I think your family genetic history' – the heart problems – 'is enough to tell that you mustn't, mustn't carry excess weight.' She had watched my fat levels creep up, and she knew that it increased my risk of illness and early death. She offered to teach me how to cook healthy meals, and to learn to dance and other fun forms of exercise. I thanked her and ignored all of it. She was thrilled when I started to take Ozempic.

I went to her one night to say I was thinking of quitting the drug, because it was not a solution to the heart of the problem. It was not dealing with the underlying causes. I was overweight because of these much bigger forces, and that was where the problem had to be tackled.

Judy was alarmed. She said: 'There is something about Britain that is causing one in every seven women to get breast cancer. That wasn't true ten years ago, twenty years ago, let alone two hundred years ago, and it isn't true in Japan. There is clearly something societally wrong – horrifyingly wrong – in this country. But, Johann, when I got breast cancer, you didn't say – "Well, fuck me, you're already in this terrible situation with cancer, and now they want to pump you full of this chemo to try to save your life? Deal with the deep societal causes of cancer instead! Let's fight for that." No. You said: "You need to do this, because in this horrible situation, it's the best option on the table for you right now." Look, Johann – I wish I lived in a country where one in seven women didn't get breast cancer. I think we should find out what the reasons are, and deal with them. But we haven't done that, and I do live in this country, and I got cancer. So I did what I had to do in order to survive it.'

Of course, she said, my excess weight wasn't as imminent a crisis as her cancer had been – but it could turn into one. 'Your weight will only keep going up unless you do something about it. I think if you lose the excess weight at your age in the way you're doing, the chances are you will lead a healthy life eating healthy food from now on. If you don't, you'll face a shorter life. And I want you around for a really long time.'

As our conversation continued, I kept returning to the anxieties expressed by Michael Lowe and the others. Judy stressed that she totally agreed with them – this is a problem with environmental causes, and we should deal with those environmental causes. We should all fight for that. It's necessary. But that's not an argument against also taking urgent remedial measures now. 'If my house is on fire, you could say, "It would be really good if we used different kinds of building materials that were less flammable and it would be really good if we could instal better sprinkler systems." Those are excellent ideas. But right now, the house is on fire. Call a fire engine, and douse the whole house in water.' She talked about how many kids at her son's school are obese, and said: 'It's at that level of crisis. I just don't see how anybody could not be in a state of complete alarm and panic about what's happening. Douse the house in water, now.'

Judy told me I had to be honest with myself. If I stopped taking the Ozempic, I would put all the weight back on, and probably it would keep piling up through the rest of my forties and fifties, and I would get sick. 'You are one of the most self-disciplined people I know. You identify goals and pursue them. You focus your efforts towards the things you care about, and you get results. But in this area of your life – changing your diet – you can't do it. It's the only area. You have really tried. I've seen how you've lost weight sometimes. It's not that you lack willpower. It's that in this world we've built, losing weight is the hardest thing in the world. Honestly, I think it's easier to give up heroin in this society than to give up all this shitty food, because at least if you stop taking heroin, you aren't in an environment where it's everywhere all around you all the time.' If I walked away from the 'effortless weight loss' of Ozempic, 'know that you are choosing a dangerous path', she said. 'Nothing is perfect, but what we've got is so catastrophically imperfect that, it feels to me, Ozempic is offering a better version of imperfection.'

~

I played over Judy's arguments in my mind for weeks, still conflicted. Then, after I spoke with a man named Jeff Parker, I thought about what she had said differently. He is a 66-year-old retired lighting designer who lives in San Francisco, and two years ago, he was obese, weighing 225 pounds. 'I was hobbled by my weight,' he said. He struggled to walk, and his legs ached horribly whenever he did. 'I tried everything. I had tried the diets, the calorie restrictions … I tried Noom and other apps. I tried calorie counting. I tried logging.' But nothing worked for long, and the effect on his health of being so overweight was terrible. His doctor told him his kidneys, liver and blood pressure were all in serious trouble, he had gout, and he was facing serious heart problems. He had to swallow fistfuls of pills every day.

Then one day, his friend Mel told him that she had been taking the weight-loss drug Mounjaro. She was increasing her dose, so she had a few 5mg pens left, and said he should try it. 'In my first month, I dropped twenty pounds,' he said. 'So the positive feedback loop started immediately.' He was able to start walking around again, and exercising a little. He told me to try carrying around a twenty-pound bag of dog food or rice for a day, everywhere I go – and then put it down. The relief I would feel is how he feels now. 'It's a weight off your shoulders. You're no longer hobbled. You can actually do the things that give you joy.' As his weight fell remarkably fast, he started to walk his little dog over the Golden Gate Bridge, strolling joyfully in the sun.

Jeff managed to get an ongoing supply of the drugs, and by the time we spoke, he had lost fifty pounds in total. His doctor was startled by his test results. 'He cut me in half on my blood pressure pills. He cut me in half on my gout pills. He cut me in half on my statin, boom! He said: "It's very likely that I'll cut you in half again on all of those drugs." All this metabolic syndrome – it's resolving. So pretty much everything that was ailing me is resolving with the weight loss. It's miraculous.' His persistent aches and pains went away. He has started to ride his bike all over the hills of San Francisco. 'I feel like I'm going to enjoy my retirement now.'

I told Jeff that I felt we should be dealing with the deeper environmental causes, and that some people think we should prioritise that over drugging people. He smiled and said: 'I think that's a good goal, and good luck with that. I'll support you with that. But I've got one life. I'm sixty-six, and I want to enjoy life now. I'm all for rebuilding the food supply, I'm all for getting sugar out of everything – it *is* in everything – but I live today, not in some future utopia where everybody grows their own kale in their yard. I live now. I need to maximise my health and my enjoyment now. Life is a finite resource.'

~

I found that hard to argue with. Daniel Drucker, who first discovered GLP-1, told me: 'While we are waiting for the magic solutions to be able to reverse our entire global epidemiology and our incidence of obesity back to where we were in the 1960s and 70s, we have something to improve health.' Dr Shauna Levy, the obesity specialist who prescribes Ozempic, said bluntly: 'Talk to the government. Talk to all of these people who have made all our foods unhealthy and our portions out of control. Go talk to them.' But 'until all those changes happen, are we not supposed to fix our man-made problem?' She waved her hand at the absurdity of this suggestion.

As I reflected more on this, I asked myself: Do you object to diabetics taking Ozempic to control their blood sugar? No. But doesn't diabetes have environmental causes? Isn't it driven, when it comes to type 2 diabetes, by the same factors that drive obesity? Yes, the evidence is clear that it is. So why are you keen for diabetics to use it to treat their environmentally triggered problem, but hesitant for obese people to take it to treat theirs?

Uncomfortably, I asked myself: Do you have this psychological objection to these drugs because, at some level, you believe that obese people don't deserve to be healthy?

This led me to confront something deeper in my psyche. If I am totally honest, at some level, I believed that by taking these drugs, I was cheating. You should get to weight loss through hard work – diet and exercise. Just being jabbed once a week is too easy. I felt slightly ashamed.

I'm not the only person who feels this way. Whenever a celebrity posts pictures of themselves on social media showing weight loss now, they are immediately accused of using Ozempic – and therefore of cheating. The Hollywood personal trainer Jono Castano, who is credited with helping the actress Rebel Wilson lose weight, said the drugs were a sign that 'people are lazy and they don't want to put in the work.'

I only really understood why I thought like this when I read about the history of how people have been taught to think about fatness. Though it was rare in the past, it did exist – and it was seen as an offence against nature. The seven deadly sins were first spelled out by Pope Gregory I in the sixth century – and one of them was gluttony. He said overeating is a sin, and sin requires punishment before you can get to redemption. It is very deep in our culture to believe that obesity is a sign a person is greedy, so suffering is the just and necessary response. The only forms of weight loss we admire are ones that involve pain – extreme exercise programmes, or extreme calorie restriction. If you go through that, we'll just about forgive you. But if you're suddenly thin at no cost in pain and sweat to you? We are outraged.

I realised I had internalised this. I felt ashamed of being fat, and at some unconscious level, I believed I deserved to be punished for it – and taking Ozempic was skipping the punishment, a get-out-of-jail free card. But when these ideas were brought to the forefront of my mind – once I had to say them out loud – I began to question them.

I thought about this more deeply when I read an essay by the Irish journalist Terry Prone, who wrote about how a similar debate had played out two hundred years ago. When modern anaesthetics were first introduced, many doctors resisted giving these painkilling options to women going through childbirth, believing that suffering was a crucial part of delivering a baby. Christ had suffered on the cross, and women should suffer when delivering a child. Suffering was ennobling. (I suspect there was also a strain of misogyny and Puritanism to it: a woman delivering a child has had sex, and that too should be followed by the infliction of pain.) To have a child without pain was cheating the laws of nature. The beliefs around this only changed very slowly. A key moment came when Queen Victoria revealed she had used anaesthetics during her childbirths. Today, few people would say that a woman was 'cheating' if she dulled the agony of childbirth with meds, and you would regard me as crazy and misogynistic if I told you that a woman giving birth deserves to suffer.

So I asked myself: why should recovering from obesity involve pain? Do I really think Jeff deserves to suffer? Or my late friend Hannah? Or my grandmother, who was obese for most of her adult life, ruining her knees and likely contributing to her dementia? Do I think they are sinners who deserve punishment – or have I moved beyond the ideas of a sixth-century pope?

One day, John Wilding – one of the scientists who played a key role in the development of these drugs – said to me: 'Why should we make it really difficult for people? Are we just punishing them?' He regarded this as a crazy idea we need to overcome. 'I say we should make it easier for them. We will then improve health.'

Unsure, unsteady, trying to process all my conflicting feelings, I decided to continue to give these drugs a chance, for now.

4

Living in an Inflamed State

What has happened to our bodies – and do these drugs reverse it?

Highly processed foods have changed our bodies and our minds, and in the short term, these drugs seem to be one of the few options available to reverse their effect on us. But the drugs clearly come with all sorts of risks of their own. So in order to think this through fully, I needed to weigh two competing forms of risk against each other. Do the risks of obesity exceed the risks of Ozempic and its sister drugs?

A big part of me didn't actually want to know what this additional weight does to your health. I felt this way for a few reasons. The first is that many of the people I love are overweight or obese, and it's frightening to be told that they are being subjected to ongoing harm by very powerful forces. The second is that the food I grew up eating is a great source of comfort and pleasure for me. I didn't want to be told that my comfort blanket might in fact be a poison. The third is that there are plenty of people out there who are hatefully cruel to overweight people, and they use the science about the dangers of obesity as a weapon against them. It's sometimes called 'concern-trolling' – where you pretend to be worried about somebody's health so you can, in fact, shame and humiliate them. I was worried that going through this evidence might inadvertently give those people ammunition.

But in the end, the argument for exploring the truth was greater than the argument to hide from it. We all know that sometimes you have to face unpleasant facts. It's tempting to hide the bill you can't pay, or to ignore the call from your doctor that might be bad news. But we open the envelope and we answer the call, because we know that if we don't, down the road, we will face a worse problem.

So I interviewed many experts about the effects on your body of being overweight or obese, and read through the best science on it in great detail. It was striking to me that there is very broad scientific agreement on the main questions. As one of Britain's best-known doctors, Max Pemberton – somebody I'll quote a lot in this chapter – told me, the scientific evidence 'shows that being overweight or obese significantly impacts on your long-term health in a number of different ways. There is absolutely no debate about it in the scientific community. The best thing you can do for your long-term health outcomes is to be within healthy weight range.'

There are a small number of activists who have tried to dispute this strong consensus. They claim that the idea obesity is harmful is a myth promoted by a medical establishment motivated by deep prejudice against fatness. In this chapter, I want to look at what the scientists say, and then in a later chapter what these activists argue in response. I approached both with an open mind.

~

The most common health effect of being overweight is the development of diabetes. I have to confess that, without giving it much thought, I had always assumed that this was a pretty minor problem. If you're diagnosed, don't you just inject yourself with insulin and bring yourself back to normal? So long as you have a regular, safe supply, isn't a diabetic's life the same as a non-diabetic's?

Max told me that lots of people think that, but as a doctor who has treated a huge number of diabetic patients, he knows that this is a catastrophic mistake. He explained how the disease works. In your pancreas, your body manufactures a hormone called insulin, which has a really important job. It helps glucose, your body's main source of energy, get into your cells. Some people naturally have a problem creating insulin, and they have type 1 diabetes. For many other people, as they become overweight, their body starts to struggle to process insulin properly, and they develop type 2 diabetes. When this happens, it means the glucose doesn't get into your cells, and key parts of your body become starved of the energy they need. This endangers your eyes, heart, kidneys and nerves. Graham MacGregor, one of Britain's leading experts on blood pressure, told me that many people 'don't realise quite what type 2 diabetes does to you'. It's one of the biggest causes of blindness in the UK. 'Biggest cause of renal dialysis. Biggest cause of bilateral leg amputation.' As a result of type 2 diabetes, every year more than 120,000 people in the US have to have lower extremities cut off.

Max said the effects of diabetes are so severe, even when it is treated well, that he has personally reached the conclusion that if he had a choice, he would rather be diagnosed as HIV-positive than diabetic. He knows that sounds shocking, but urged me to look at the facts. 'This is from a purely medical point of view. At the moment, people with HIV [who receive treatment] are living as long as somebody without. Someone with diabetes? You lose fifteen years of your life on average,' if you get it as a young adult. And it's not just that you die much earlier. You are far more likely to live with terrible complications, often for years. 'If you look at the last few years of your life with diabetes,' the odds are significantly increased that you 'may be quite severely disabled. You might be blind. You might have renal failure. These are the complications of diabetes ... You might have your leg amputated. You might have a stroke, so you're paralysed down one side. You might have vascular dementia. There are multiple things that could affect you if you have diabetes before it kills you.'

An obese man is six times more likely to develop diabetes than a non-obese man, and an obese woman is twelve times more likely. A scientific overview looking at 2.3 million individuals with type 2 diabetes found 'a strong positive linear' association between body mass and diabetes – as your body mass goes up, so does your risk of diabetes. If your BMI is over 35 when you are eighteen years old, you have an over 70 per cent chance of becoming diabetic at some point in your life.

It's shockingly easy to start on this path. In a simple experiment, a team of scientists took six healthy men and got them to just lie in bed and eat 6,000 calories a day. Within forty-eight hours, they had developed insulin resistance, the first step to diabetes. It's now very common: more than a third of the US population is currently in a pre-diabetic state, where their blood sugar levels are getting out of control because of some insulin resistance, while 12 to 14 per cent have gone into full-blown diabetes.

The next most common effect of gaining weight is an increase in physical pain. It strains your back, your knees, your hips. At my fattest – when I was fifteen stone in my late twenties – I remember a stabbing pain in my lower back that kept me awake at night. The fatter you get, the more this limits your ability to live a full life. A few years ago, I went to visit the Grand Canyon. It was a seven-hour drive in a minibus from Vegas, and in my little tour group, there was a very funny and charming nine-year-old boy. He was brimming with facts about the Canyon, which he had been learning all about at school. He was also severely obese. When we arrived, the driver dropped us off, and we were due to walk along the perimeter of the Canyon for a mile or so and meet up with him again further down. About halfway there, this bright little boy was breathless, covered with sweat, and said his feet hurt so much that he couldn't walk any more. He wasn't staring at the Canyon in awe. He was almost in tears, and his parents, themselves breathless, looked humiliated and ashamed. They called the coach driver, and he came as close as he could to pick them up.

As you get older, carrying this excess weight damages your knees and hips, because of simple wear and tear. 'It's just because of the sheer weight you're putting through your limbs,' Max told me. When your legs carry more weight, your cartilage gets corroded. This is why if you're an overweight man, you are 176 per cent more likely to need to have a knee or hip replaced, and if you're obese, the odds go up by 320 per cent.

Another major effect of being overweight is that it endangers your heart. This felt very close to home for me, because – as I mentioned before – it's what killed my grandfather when he was slightly younger than I am now. Max explained that there are several ways it does this. 'Your heart pumps blood around your body – but in itself, it's a muscle. It needs its own supply of blood.' Obesity 'causes narrowing of the blood vessels that supply your heart'. Over time, this can mean 'your heart doesn't have enough blood going through it. Then you get angina. It gets almost like a cramp, because it's not getting enough oxygen.' Separately, gaining weight 'increases your blood pressure, which affects your heart. It increases your risk of atherosclerosis, because plaques form in your blood vessels, which can then lead you to have a heart attack.' For every five-unit increase in BMI, your chance of heart failure goes up by 41 per cent. This problem is rising as obesity rises: the number of Americans whose death from heart disease was attributed by doctors to obesity tripled between 1999 and 2020.

Max and I went down the list of illnesses we all fear most – stroke and cancer, for example – and he showed me that the scientific evidence suggests they hugely increase in likelihood as you gain weight. A meta-analysis covering over 2 million people found that 'overweight and obese individuals had, respectively, 22 per cent and 64 per cent greater probability of an ischemic stroke compared with normal-weight subjects'. Graham MacGregor told me: 'It's one thing doctors worry about – getting a stroke, and surviving. Paralysed. Unable to speak for the rest of your life. You may live another five or ten years, totally dependent on other people. Absolute nightmare.'

'Most people don't realise that obesity is closely linked to cancer,' Max said, but in fact, between 4 and 8 per cent of cancers are attributable to obesity, and it is the second biggest cause of cancer in countries like the US and Britain. A large meta-analysis found 'strong evidence' linking obesity to not just one but nine different types of cancer. The leading British cancer charity, Cancer Research UK, explains: 'If you are overweight you are more likely to get cancer than if you are a healthy weight … Being overweight doesn't mean that you'll definitely develop cancer. But the risk is higher the more overweight you are and the longer you are overweight for … Extra fat in the body doesn't just sit there, it's active and sends out signals to the rest of your body. These signals can tell cells in our body to divide more often, which can lead to cancer.' In addition, it can cause inflammation, which causes cells to divide more quickly.

This concept – inflammation – is, I learned, crucial for understanding a lot of the harm that happens to you as you gain weight. Dr Giles Yeo, the obesity researcher at Cambridge University, told me that whenever your body is injured, the injured area becomes inflamed. Cut your finger, and it becomes swollen and inflamed for a while. This is a crucial part of the healing process – inflammation is the alert signal that tells your body there's a problem, so it can send emergency resources to the damaged area in order to nurse it back to health. When the injury heals, the inflammation goes away. But, Giles said, obesity seems to screw with this process, for a simple reason. As you gain weight, your fat cells expand, but they can only go so far. 'As your fat cells begin to reach the limit of their ability to expand, your body senses the stretch as damage.' Because it knows something is wrong, your body floods the area with inflammation – but this time, because the stretching doesn't go away, the inflammation doesn't go away. When this happens, your body's healing processes can go haywire. Your immune system can't repair damage properly any more. The processes that are meant to heal you start to hurt you. The fire brigade turns into the fire. This is one reason for the increased cancer risks, and many of the other dangers obese people face.

I felt slightly numbed as I realised that the negative effects of being overweight or obese go on and on. They make it more likely you'll develop asthma, sleep apnoea (where you don't breathe properly in your sleep, and always wake up feeling exhausted), arthritis, kidney problems, fertility problems, gallstones, thrombosis and – for me perhaps the most frightening of all – dementia.

There are, to balance against this, a small number of health benefits of being overweight or obese. For example, you are less likely to break a bone or to develop osteoporosis than people of a normal or lower weight, because carrying all that weight gives you a workout and makes your bones stronger. There is a very strong scientific consensus, however, that the risks of being overweight are significant and outweigh these relatively small benefits. A large study by the US National Cancer Institute followed half a million Americans for ten years, and found that if you are overweight, your chances of dying of any cause in the next ten years increase by 20 to 40 per cent. If you are obese, they increase by 200 to 300 per cent.

As I spoke to the scientists who made these bleak discoveries, I was struck by how many of them had lost their parents young. Often, they had been killed by the very conditions they were now trying to warn the world about. Graham's father died of a heart attack when he was in his fifties. Tim Spector lost his dad to a heart condition when his father was just fifty-seven. It was clear to me they are not driven by prejudice. They are driven by love, and a desire to prevent suffering.

~

When you look at this evidence without flinching, the argument for these drugs becomes obvious. Perhaps the best comparison group is people who have gone through bariatric surgery. They all start off obese, and on average, after surgery, they lose 27.5 per cent of their body weight, which is only a little more than the most cutting-edge weight-loss drugs are producing in clinical trials. So I wanted to know: what else, if anything, changes in their health following this dramatic weight loss?

The findings are startling. Seventy-five per cent of the people who had diabetes see it vanish entirely. Sixty per cent of the patients who had hypertension see it disappear. There is a huge reduction in physical pain: one study found that for two-thirds of people with back pain, it totally goes away. But it is the results with the deadly diseases that are most striking. After bariatric surgery, a study of over 15,000 people found the chance of dying from diabetes falls by 92 per cent, of dying from cancer falls by 60 per cent, and of dying of coronary heart disease falls by 56 per cent. These effects are so dramatic that in the seven years after the operation, for people who had been severely obese, the chance of dying *of any cause* falls by 40 per cent.

Bariatric surgery is a drastic intervention, with a lot of downsides. It involves having large parts of your insides removed, and around one in a thousand people who have it die during the operation or of complications later. Afterwards, your stomach is smaller, and if you try to eat more than a limited amount, you become very uncomfortable. For a small but significant minority, it can lead to serious psychological problems – ones I'll explore later, because they may pose a parallel warning for these drugs. I am not making the case for or against this kind of surgery. But the massive overall improvement in health that people experience after bariatric surgery does prove an important point: if you successfully reverse obesity, you reverse most of the health harms I have described in this chapter. This means you do not have to be permanently locked into much higher odds of diabetes, cancer, dementia and death.

Scientists are starting to find similar health improvements in people who use the new weight-loss drugs. In August 2023, we learned the results of the first major study into how using Wegovy (the same drug as Ozempic, but marketed for obese people instead of diabetics) affects health over the medium term. For five years, a group of scientists working for the pharmaceutical company Novo Nordisk followed 17,000 adults over the age of forty-five who had a BMI of 27 or higher. Some were given a placebo, and some were given the real drug, and the changes in their health were tracked. By the end of the study, the people who got the real drug were 20 per cent less likely to have a heart attack and 20 per cent less likely to have a stroke. It lowered their blood pressure, reduced the amount of inflammation in their bodies, and positively changed the balance of the lipids in their blood. Indeed, it improved people's health on twenty-eight different measures, including kidney disease.

We need to be cautious here, because this is a study from the drug company itself, and it has yet to be published in a peer-reviewed journal. But it was carried out by serious scientists who know it will soon be published and scrutinised, and it is a staggering finding. If it is borne out, it means that using these drugs, we could prevent one in five of the heart attacks or strokes that affect overweight or obese people. That would save 1.5 million lives across a decade in the US alone.

That's what you get if you take Wegovy, which on average reduces obesity in individuals by 10 to 15 per cent. What will we see from the next generation of these drugs, which are poised to reduce obesity by as much as 30 per cent?

When I told a friend about these findings, he said, 'Wow, this drug has amazing effects – it's like magic.' But I told him that it's not that the drug produces all of these twenty-eight different effects on people. It's that obesity produces an extraordinary amount of harm, across all sorts of measures – and the drug primarily does one thing: it slashes obesity. That's why it seems to have such an incredibly broad array of effects.

For all my doubts about the drugs, I had to stop and acknowledge this. For the first time in my research for this book, I felt a real thrill of excitement. Given the history of heart disease in my family, it could save my life. I thought back over all the people I know who have experienced the negative effects of obesity – such as my friend Hannah, dead at forty-six, or an elderly friend of mine who is in agony with her knees and is almost trapped in her home now because she can't get up and down stairs. It's too late for them – but could this turn around the lives of people like them? Could it save that little boy, who longed to see the Grand Canyon, but couldn't even walk alongside it for more than a few minutes?

~

The advantages of these drugs were now clear to me. That's one side of the ledger. So now I needed to investigate – what are the risks? Can you really get such huge benefits without paying a cost? Can it all be so easy?

5

An Old Story Repeating Itself?

The risks of the old weight-loss drugs – and the new ones

In the twentieth century, a pattern emerged. A new miracle weight-loss drug was announced by scientists. People started taking it and discovered that it really worked. They shed weight. Then more and more people took it – until a fatal flaw was discovered in the drug, and it had to be withdrawn from the market. Then there would be disillusionment about diet drugs for a decade. But then another miracle drug would be announced, and the tango would start all over again. So even when I ran my hand over my flattening stomach, I wondered: What if all this is just an old story, repeating itself?

The tale of modern diet drugs began in a French factory at the height of the First World War, when a weird accident took place. Men who were building munitions using an explosive yellow powder named dinitrophenol noticed that they had started to lose weight rapidly. It turned out they were absorbing the explosive both through their skin and by breathing it in, and this was causing them to lose their appetites. A group of American scientists at Stanford University heard about this, and began to research the potential of the explosive as a weight-loss drug. They discovered that people who took it as a pill lost two pounds a week effortlessly, without feeling at all hungry. They then uncovered the mechanism that made it work: if you took it, your metabolism would speed up by between 30 and 50 per cent.

The drug companies of the day seized on this and started to market the chemical as Redusols, 'a new and safe way to lose weight' and an 'anti-obesity therapy'. It became wildly popular, especially when you bear in mind that obesity was so much lower than it is today. By 1934, 100,000 people were taking it. But then people started to notice the drug had other effects. If you took a low dose, you would often sweat profusely, or lose your sense of taste. If you took a medium dose, you often developed cataracts and went blind. The drug worked in part by raising your body temperature – it was, after all, an explosive – and doctors began to realise with horror that if you used it at a high dose, it could literally cook you from the inside. The historian Hillel Schwartz explains that for heavy users 'there is a fatal hyperpyremia. That is, the body succumbs to an extraordinarily high fever. It burns itself up.' By 1938, Redusols was banned. It continued for years to be used as a powerful pesticide, because it is so good at killing anything that lives.

A few years later, there was another breakthrough. American soldiers in the Second World War were often given amphetamine pills to keep them alert during boring but essential tasks, like watching radar for approaching enemy ships. They too lost a lot of weight. Once the war was over, these pills were quickly marketed as a treatment for the overweight that was targeted particularly at women. It was known as 'mother's little helper', because it had a double benefit: these pills dramatically suppressed your appetite, and at the same time, they gave you a huge boost of energy, making you manically active. These pills were so wildly popular that by 1952, around 2 billion of them were manufactured for the weight-loss market alone. By the summer of 1970, 8 per cent of all prescriptions in the US were for amphetamines.

But if you take lots of amphetamines over a significant period of time, you develop something called tolerance. Dr Robert Kushner, who has prescribed these drugs in the past, told me: 'People would often say, "[They don't] work as well any more." If you know anyone addicted to amphetamines, you have to take higher and higher doses for the same high. I think the same thing probably occurs here.' Your body gets used to the drugs. This meant that typically, when you took them, you lost a lot of weight in the first six to ten weeks, but then you had a choice: either stay at the current dose and see your weight come back, or jack up the dose of the drug you take. People soon discovered that increasing the drug brings problems of its own: as your dose gets higher, you become much more likely to experience paranoia, anxiety, psychosis and damage to your heart. In the early 1970s, one of the first big crusades of the 'Fat Pride' movement – a group of fat people who banded together to fight back against stigma and discrimination – was to warn that taking these pills was dangerous and people shouldn't be pressured to take them. They were vindicated. As many people became addicted or went crazy, these amphetamine-based weight-loss drugs became severely restricted.

A few can still be prescribed in the US for weight loss. Shauna Levy, who reluctantly prescribes one of them, told me: 'Most patients lose weight up front, but long term, they don't seem to be able to keep the weight off.' It makes their hearts race and they feel anxious. 'Some people have an increase in their blood pressure, headaches, not [being] able to sleep.' The only benefit is they are 'pretty cheap, so you can just do cash pay' if you don't have insurance or your insurance doesn't cover it. 'I know it's their only option' for financial reasons, but 'when I look at the patients in front of me, it's never really felt like a great option'.

~

In their place, in the 1970s a series of bizarre alternatives began to grow in popularity. One was known as the 'Sleeping Beauty Diet'. It was based on a madly simple idea: if you're unconscious, you can't eat. People began to take sleeping pills that kept them unconscious for twenty hours a day, or even got put into medically induced comas. It produced lots of sleeping pill addictions, and no lasting weight loss.

Perhaps the most horrific 'treatment' was jaw-wiring. This was when a dentist would attach a metal bracket to the top and bottom rows of your teeth, and then wire them shut, so that only a tiny space remained. The idea was that then you wouldn't be able to cram food into your mouth any more, and you would be forced to eat less. You would also struggle to speak, or brush your teeth, or consume anything that wasn't in liquid form. It was quickly discovered that if you vomited while your jaw was wired shut, you could easily choke to death. Still, some doctors continued doing this to people for years. Invariably, when your jaw-wiring 'treatment' ended after six months, you would regain the weight you had lost, and be horribly traumatised.

~

The next big diet drug 'breakthrough' came in the 1990s with the announcement of something called fen-phen, which combined two sets of chemicals that had been around for years. Scientists had known about an appetite suppressant named flexfluramine for a while, and there was no doubt that it successfully slashed people's hunger – but there was a drawback: it also made people very drowsy, so it wasn't much use on its own. So a scientist decided to try combining it with phentermine. He figured it would be a win-win: the amphetamine would counteract the sleepiness caused by the appetite suppressant, and it would also suppress appetite in its own right. When he gave it to 120 obese people, he found it was incredibly successful. The average person lost thirty pounds.

Based on this small study, it was announced by the drug company producing it that a cure for obesity had been found, and the media swallowed the hype. *Time* magazine ran a cover story entitled 'The New Miracle Drug?' It blew up. By 1995, there were 18 million fen-phen prescriptions in the United States alone. People were told by the drug companies there were 'no bad effects … just dizziness, maybe you get a little dry mouth. Maybe you get a little drowsy.'

It worked extraordinarily well, triggering huge levels of weight loss across the US. Many people who took the drug felt they had finally been freed from their lifelong enslavement to overeating. Richard Atkinson, who directed the Obtech Obesity Research Center, explained back then: 'Everybody who ever treated obese people and put them on fen-phen had a patient say to them, "I felt normal for the first time."' It's not that they were able to use their willpower to resist doughnuts, the patients kept saying – it's that, often for the first time in their lives, they didn't want doughnuts in the first place.

Mary Linnen was a typical person taking the drug, and her story was captured by the brilliant investigative journalist Alicia Mundy in her book *Dispensing with the Truth*. Mary was a woman from Massachusetts in her late twenties, and as soon as she got engaged, she decided she needed to lose twenty-five pounds for her wedding day. Her doctor prescribed fen-phen. Eleven days later, she was walking up a hill with her parents when she suddenly said: 'I can't breathe. I think I'm going to faint.' Everyone thought it was just some passing problem – a bug, maybe. But the sickness didn't go away, and twenty-three days later, she went to her doctor, who told her to stop taking the drug. Even then, the awful physical sensations didn't pass. Climbing the stairs left her feeling totally exhausted, and she had bouts of chest pain. Eventually, she was diagnosed with primary pulmonary hypertension, a disorder where the blood vessels in your lungs narrow, and a huge amount of pressure builds up inside them. She was told she'd have to be hooked up to an oxygen machine for the rest of her life, and that she could never have kids.

Mary told her fiancé Tom he didn't have to go through with marrying her. He replied by buying her a wedding ring.

Then one day not long after, while she was going through guest lists for their wedding, she said: 'Something's wrong. I can't breathe.' In the ambulance, she told Tom she was terrified of dying, and begged him to find a way to save her. She died a few hours later.

Fen-phen, it turned out, caused two very serious health problems. If you took it, you were around thirty times more likely to develop primary pulmonary hypertension, and it also caused heart defects in around a third of the people who used it. These effects were not disclosed to the world by the drug companies, or by the drug regulators. They were spotted by ordinary doctors in the town of Fargo, North Dakota, who became worried that so many of their patients seemed to be getting heart problems after taking it, and raised a safety signal, saying this had to be investigated.

When investigators pursued the question of how such a dangerous drug ever got to market, it emerged that both the companies and the regulator had good reason to be aware of these risks all along. As Alicia Mundy reported, a consultant employed by one of the companies had 'pinpointed valve disease' as a risk early on, and another of the companies said in an internal memo: 'If we tell what we know … that will really bring doctors' attention to the risk of primary pulmonary hypertension … It's going to have an effect on the bottom line.' In another internal email, one of the administrators wrote: 'Can I look forward to my waning years signing checks for fat people who are a little afraid of some silly lung problem?'

Finally, it was revealed that when the regulators at the Food and Drug Administration had initially considered the drug, their committee voted by five to three to reject it – precisely because of these safety concerns, according to a subsequent investigation by the *New York Times*. Their own internal memos had indicated that there were 'real concerns … about the pulmonary hypertension issue'. But after the committee voted not to allow it onto the market, one member made an appeal to the rest. He said that obesity causes so much harm to health that they needed to approve this drug. Moved by his eloquence, the others changed their minds, and voted to approve.

The companies and doctors responsible for these drugs have had to pay out more than $12 billion to the thousands of people they seriously harmed – the largest pharmaceutical settlement in history up to that point.

After learning all this, I thought: What are the chances that, in a decade or so, we'll be talking about the new weight-loss drugs like this?

~

There are fundamental differences between what happened then and what is happening now. As the later investigations revealed, fen-phen was recklessly rushed to market based on a single small study, whereas the new weight-loss drugs have undergone rigorous testing and are manufactured by some of the most reputable companies in the world. The new weight-loss drugs also work through a totally different set of mechanisms, one that has been proven in dozens of clinical trials.

But there is – in one narrow sense – a way in which, in a worst-case scenario, there might be something to learn from the fen-phen debacle when it comes to the new drugs. As with all pharmaceutical drugs, there is an inherent long-term risk. This is because most drugs brought to market are tested for short-term safety only. With fen-phen, the real benefits to health that these drugs delivered by causing significant weight loss were outweighed in the medium to longer term by harms that few people saw coming. Given the lack of long-term research in using the new generations of weight-loss drugs to treat obese people, it seems legitimate to ask – is it possible to glimpse any forms of harm now that could be harbingers of worse to come?

This isn't a dilemma that's unique to the new weight-loss drugs, and it isn't the fault of the drug companies. It is standard practice with the release of new drugs. The drug companies are behaving properly within the existing rules and regulations. But usually, a new drug has a slow roll-out, so medium-term risks can begin to be identified by doctors and public health officials before huge numbers of people take them. Fen-phen showed us that with a new diet drug, there can easily be a stampede to use it, because people are so desperate to lose weight, and the moment they find something that works, huge numbers of people want it. So we go from zero people using a new drug to hundreds of thousands or even millions of people taking it in a very short space of time. This can mean that by the time you spot a long-term risk using the normal methods of doctors or public health officials flagging them up, it has affected a large number of people.

Many of the scientists I spoke with said there is one reason, above all others, why we should be broadly confident that these drugs are safe. Diabetics have been taking them for a long time now – and it hasn't caused any unexpected effects to them. Speaking in April 2023, Daniel Drucker, the man who discovered GLP-1, told me: 'We've had literally millions of lives exposed to these drugs now over the past eighteen years' since GLP-1 agonists were first licensed as medicines for diabetes, and 'if you actually look in the real-world databases of countries that record who's on what drug and what are their outcomes … there's no safety signal. None.' This means no doctors have observed their patients getting sick beyond the well-known side effects.

Daniel added a caveat to this. It's important to acknowledge, he said, that these are people taking the drug for diabetes, not obesity. So 'it is correct to say we don't have the same database yet for people who are losing weight and do not have type 2 diabetes'. It could affect obese people differently from how it affects diabetics. 'As a scientist, you respect the gaps in our evidence.' But he has a high level of confidence that if these drugs had significant unknown negative effects, they would have emerged in the large diabetic populations taking them by now. Most of the scientists I spoke to agreed. These drugs have been subject to extensive and rigorous trials, and have been in use in a parallel population for years. It's an important point, and it's one that gives many people confidence in the drugs.

But a smaller number of scientists and doctors said that while this is likely a correct point, there's a reason to hesitate. Max Pemberton told me he doesn't take as much comfort from the fact that diabetics have been taking them for a long time, for one reason. 'That's a cohort of people who are already unwell.' Indeed, they have a degenerative condition, and they get sicker over time. So it could be easy for Ozempic to be causing some negative effect on diabetics and for that to be missed by doctors, because they would assume it's simply part of the general worsening of health experienced by many diabetics. For example, Max said, imagine if Ozempic made people more likely to be depressed. That could easily be missed, because 'people with chronic health conditions are already more likely to be depressed'.

~

As I studied the evidence that's emerging slowly, I learned that there are twelve potential risks that could be associated with these new weight-loss drugs. (I'll talk about ten of them in this chapter, and two will emerge later in the book.)

The first two are by far the most trivial, but they trouble some people. These drugs can cause such rapid weight loss that both your face and your buttocks can start to look deflated and saggy. This has become known as 'Ozempic face' and 'Ozempic butt'. To treat the rush of gaunt faces that have emerged, there's a stampede for fillers to be injected into people's faces. There's no physical risk here – just an aesthetic one. I have to confess I was never worried about this. I have such a naturally fat, round face that every single baby I ever encounter smiles at me immediately: I think they believe I am their king. My face could deflate a long way without ever looking sunken. But for other people, it can be upsetting.

The third is far more serious. A few months after Daniel told me there was no safety signal attached to these drugs, one was raised for the first time. The European Medicines Agency – the regulatory body for the European Union – announced 'a thyroid cancer safety signal' for all GLP-1 agonists. This means that they were beginning to monitor the drugs for potentially causing thyroid cancer. They did this because of a worrying piece of research that was published in France by Jean-Luc Faillie, who is a professor of medical pharmacology at the University Hospital of Montpellier and also in charge of the National Pharmacovigilance Survey of these drugs for the French Medicine Agency. He told me that for several years it's been known that when GLP-1 agonists are given to rats and mice 'they have shown an increased risk of thyroid cancer'. It is also known that human beings 'have GLP-1 receptors in their thyroid tissue', so it's conceivable that messing with GLP-1 might mess with your thyroid.

So Jean-Luc decided he and his team needed to dig into this. France has one of the largest medical databases in the world, so they went back and analysed the data for all the patients with type 2 diabetes who had taken these drugs for one to three years, in the period between 2006 and 2018. They then compared those patients to a sample of diabetics who had not taken these drugs. Their findings were startling. He said bluntly: 'We show there is an increased risk of about 50 to 75 per cent more' of you developing thyroid cancer.

He told me it's important not to misread this. This doesn't mean that if you take the drug, you have a 50 to 75 per cent chance of developing thyroid cancer. It means that if you take the drug, your chances will be 50 to 75 per cent higher than they would have been had you not taken the drug. Nonetheless, this seemed to me to be a disturbing increase. In most of the commentary on this study, it was repeatedly argued that it was a low risk. I said to Jean-Luc that maybe I was being dumb, but those figures don't seem low to me. 'Yeah. It's not low,' he said. 'In epidemiology in general, when you have a 50 per cent increase, it's quite a thing.' But then he explained why many scientists would still reasonably continue to describe this as a low risk. 'The incidence of thyroid cancer is very low. It's not a very frequent cancer.' (Currently, around 1.2 per cent of people will get thyroid cancer in their lifetimes, and 84 per cent of them survive it.) 'So if you increase [levels by] 50 per cent, there is an increased incidence, but it remains low.' But he added: 'Given the exposure [of these drugs] to millions of patients, there will be some cases of thyroid cancer that maybe we could avoid.'

The FDA (Food and Drug Administration) in the US advises people with a family history of thyroid cancer not to use these drugs, and Jean-Luc argues that the European regulators should do the same. The European Medicines Agency took several months to review the evidence that he and other scientists presented, and concluded that the limited evidence that is available 'does not support a causal relationship' between GLP-1 agonists and thyroid cancer in humans. They urged the companies involved to continue to monitor the data on this as it evolves. Jean-Luc told me that with all medical interventions, you have to balance risks and benefits, and he believes this risk around thyroid cancer should be explained to people clearly so they can make an informed choice. If you are diabetic or severely obese, he said, the benefits outweigh the risks. 'But in the case of slightly overweight patients, who take the drug for more aesthetic benefits,' in his view, it's not worth the risk.

~

The fourth risk is to your pancreas, which is the organ that helps you to digest food by releasing digestive enzymes. Taking GLP-1 agonists can have an effect on the pancreatic cells that produce these enzymes, causing them to go haywire. I spoke with Michelle Stesiak, a woman in her fifties from Myrtle Beach in South Carolina. When she started taking Ozempic, she asked her doctor if there were any risks, and she said there were none, except a very slight chance of a condition named pancreatitis, where your pancreas becomes dangerously inflamed. Michelle laughed and said, 'Oh, knowing me, I'll get it.' She took the drug for six weeks and was very happy with the results, and then she flew to Pittsburgh to visit her daughter.

She woke up at three in the morning and 'I thought I was dying. It was the most excruciating pain I've ever experienced.' She felt a strip of searing agony running from under her breasts, all the way around her left side, to her back, and 'I was immediately in the foetal position. I couldn't speak. I was vomiting profusely and I had full-blown diarrhoea.' Her son-in-law called an ambulance. At the hospital, 'you couldn't touch my stomach – even a blanket touching it was excruciating'. They gave her fentanyl for the pain and tried to figure out what had happened. At first, they thought her bowels were twisted, but then her tests showed something different: her pancreas was in serious trouble. They asked her if she was a heavy drinker. She said no. They asked her if she'd had gallstones. She said no. Then they asked her if she was taking Ozempic.

Michelle quit the drug, and within a month, she had made a full recovery, but she told me the pain she'd experienced was much worse than any of her childbirths. Doctors often compare the pain of pancreatitis to being stabbed with a knife. Michelle was confident that if she hadn't received urgent medical care, she would have died. She said that people taking Ozempic need to know 'it can cause pancreatitis, and very quickly. It's something you don't want to mess around with.'

A group of Canadian scientists at the University of British Columbia analysed health data for people taking semaglutide (Ozempic and Wegovy) and similar drugs between 2006 and 2020, and found that if you take them, you are nine times more likely to get pancreatitis. That still meant it was 'rare' – but it's a considerable rise in risk. According to the NHS, four out of five cases of pancreatitis go away when they are treated and don't cause any long-term problems – but for the others, it can cause serious problems, including in very extreme cases organ failure and death.

~

The fifth risk is that you could develop a condition known as 'stomach paralysis'. This is an unusual condition where your digestive system slows down and your body struggles to move food from your stomach to your small intestine. In extreme cases, your stomach can become frozen, with the food trapped and rotting inside you. The same group of Canadian scientists found that these new weight-loss drugs increase the odds of stomach paralysis by 3.67 times. Similarly, the risk of developing a bowel obstruction goes up by 4.22 times. A 44-year-old woman from Louisiana is suing both Novo Nordisk and Eli Lilly, claiming that she was insufficiently warned about this risk, and that after taking Ozempic and then Mounjaro, she suffered a paralysed stomach and the condition made her vomit so violently that she lost teeth. Her lawyers say they are investigating 400 other potential cases like this. Another woman named Brea Hand (who isn't involved in the court case) told CBS News that when she developed stomach paralysis while taking Ozempic 'the stomach pain was just unbearable and I couldn't keep anything down. I would drink something and within minutes, like five, ten minutes later, I would be throwing up.' The companies involved are disputing these legal cases vigorously.

~

The sixth risk is to your muscle mass. This is the total amount of soft muscle tissue you have in your body, and it has to be at the right level for you to be able to move around and for you to be able to carry out basic bodily functions. Whenever you lose a lot of weight – whether it's by dieting, or illness, or exercise – you usually lose muscle mass. So Heath Schmidt, the head of the Lab of Neuropsychopharmacology at Penn State University, told me: 'You're not just losing fat when you're on these drugs. Some individuals are also losing 20 to 30 per cent lean [muscle] mass, which in the long term could be problematic.' He looked concerned. 'You don't want to lose muscle mass ever, but that seems to be one of the components of this weight loss that we're seeing.'

If your muscle mass falls too far, this can cause you serious problems as you age. Everybody naturally loses some muscle mass as they get older. After the age of thirty, it begins to decline by around 8 per cent a decade, and after you turn sixty, that process accelerates further. If your muscle mass falls too far, you will be physically weaker and less mobile. You become more likely to fall, and if you do, you are more likely to break or fracture a bone. Falling is already the biggest cause of accidental death among people aged over sixty-five – so more falls means more death. You are also more likely to develop a condition called sarcopenia (which in Greek means 'poverty of the flesh'), where your muscle mass is so low that you are left frail, vulnerable and less able to carry out normal daily tasks like climbing the stairs. This currently affects 25 per cent of elderly people. People who are already thin, who are taking this drug to become super-thin, will be particularly at risk, because they have less muscle mass to lose in the first place.

To some degree, this danger can be counterbalanced by pairing the drugs with a lot of strength and resistance training, to keep your muscle mass up. It's why I continued to go to a personal trainer twice a week and stepped up my (admittedly pitifully weak) weightlifting, and I was relieved to see that six months after starting Ozempic, my muscle mass had held steady. But I'm in my forties. That would have been harder to achieve in my seventies. For older people considering taking these drugs, the risk of sarcopenia should be carefully considered when they are calculating whether it is worth it. For younger people, they should realise that while there are big health benefits now, there may be costs further down the road.

Revealingly, it seems the drug companies themselves are concerned about this. Eli Lilly, who manufacture Mounjaro, are testing giving people semaglutide in combination with a drug that preserves muscle mass as you lose weight.

~

The seventh risk is malnutrition. A relative of mine started to take one of the weight-loss drugs not long after I did, and after a few months, I became really worried about her. She was eating very little, and was tired and unwell a lot of the time. Her kids and I often had to remind her to eat something. These drugs – especially in high doses – can dial down your appetite so dramatically that you cease to get the nutrients you need to be healthy. When you have malnutrition, you are tired and lethargic all the time, you are more likely to become depressed, you find it hard to focus, you are more likely to become sick, and if you are injured, it will take your body longer to heal. It was disconcertingly predictable that these drugs would have this effect. After bariatric surgery, malnutrition is quite common, and half of the people who have it need to be on nutritional supplements for the rest of their lives. It is something that people need to be warned about. Some doctors, when they prescribe these drugs, are now also 'prescribing' a specific diet for them to eat with a floor of calorie consumption that they mustn't fall below, to make sure their patients don't plunge too far.

~

The eighth and ninth risks stem not from the drugs themselves, but from the huge demand for them – and what it has made some of us do to get them. Shortly before I started taking Ozempic, it was clear there was going to be a massive worldwide rush for these drugs. The drug companies worked very hard to keep up with demand – but it was increasingly obvious it would take years to scale up production to meet this level. As a result, there wasn't going to be enough for everyone. In a sensible society, we would have replicated what Britain did with the Covid-19 vaccine, and rationed it according to need. We gave it to the oldest and most vulnerable people first, and the youngest and least at risk last. With these new drugs, we should have put diabetics and severely overweight people first in line, and people like me towards the back of the queue. That didn't happen. Instead, there was a scramble, and in the shoving, some of the people with the greatest need were deprived of the drug.

Zami Jalil is a 41-year-old musician who has played with one of my favourite bands, Pulp, and when I spoke with him in the spring of 2023, he was really distressed. He has type 2 diabetes, and as soon as he had started to take Ozempic a few years before, his blood sugar levels stabilised, his energy levels went up, and 'I just started to feel better' across the board. He realised he could stave off the drastic step of having to take insulin daily, a gruelling and unpleasant process that it's hard to come back from. He was thrilled. But one day, he went to his local pharmacy, and they told him that they might be about to run out of Ozempic. It was only then, he said, that he learned 'people see it as a miracle jab and therefore they're just taking it as a quick fix to lose weight'. He could understand why people want it for that purpose – but they should wait until people with greater need are safely covered. In this situation, 'you're taking it away from those with diabetes.' He became impassioned and said: 'Having elevated blood sugar, even for a few weeks, reduces your life expectancy' if you are diabetic. 'So actually, you're really killing us.'

I didn't have the courage to tell him that I was one of those people. I told myself that if I hadn't bought the Ozempic pen stashed in my fridge, it would have been bought by somebody else seeking weight loss, and given the market dynamics, that's probably true – but only in the narrowest sense. If people like me, as a group, hadn't put our own needs ahead of the greater needs of diabetics as a group, then Zami and the others like him wouldn't have been facing that pain. I could have told him about the history of heart disease in my family, and that these drugs cut cardiac events by 20 per cent – but I knew even then, his need was greater. I felt ashamed.

The next risk emerged when many people who couldn't get the branded Ozempic turned to buying off-brand knock-offs, the chemical equivalent of a fake Louis Vuitton handbag. These were either being brewed in beauty shops and spas or ordered online. Jeff Parker, the guy in San Francisco who lost a huge amount of weight, and saw a massive improvement in his health, told me that he initially got on-brand Mounjaro, but when his insurance wouldn't cover the cost of $350 a week, he decided to take a drastic step. He banded together with a group of people he met on an internet forum, and ordered an off-brand compound from a factory in China for $50 a week. It comes as a crystallised powder, with a vial of water that you have to mix in a syringe. With each new batch, one of the people on the forum pays to have it tested in a US lab – at the cost of another $300 – to make sure it is pure and not contaminated. Jeff said he has worries, of course: 'Anything coming out of a non-FDA-approved lab is concerning.' But he sees the choice as either the Chinese knock-off or ongoing obesity, with all the harm that does.

Robert Kushner, the doctor who has been a central part of developing the drug, says this is horribly alarming. He has had patients who come to him taking these compounded versions of the drugs, and 'I have no idea what's in it. I talk to patients and I have to bite my tongue not to make them feel self-conscious. I'll say "Do you know what's in it? Do you know what the dosage is?" And they say "No, no." I'm thinking in my head – how stupid can you be? You're injecting something, and you don't even know what it is.' I asked him what the risk is. 'I have no idea what it is. The risk is that I don't know what the risk is, because it's not the drug.' This kind of *Breaking Bad* Ozempic could, he said, be literally anything. In Austria in October 2023, several people bought what they believed to be Ozempic from a knock-off retailer, and suddenly started to have seizures. The hospitals they were admitted to discovered they had been taking a totally different drug.

Shauna Levy, who prescribes Ozempic in Louisiana, told me that whenever you buy a bootleg version of these weight-loss drugs, the most you can hope is that 'maybe' they are safe. 'But are you willing to risk your life on a maybe?'

~

The tenth risk might seem more hazy at first. After 9/11, the US Secretary of Defense, Donald Rumsfeld, famously said the US faced several different categories of risk: 'There are known knowns. These are things we know that we know. There are known unknowns. That is to say, there are things that we know we don't know. But there are also unknown unknowns. There are things we don't know we don't know.' With these weight-loss drugs, there are known unknowns, relating to thyroid cancer, loss of muscle mass and malnutrition, where we aren't sure yet of their scale. But there are also unknown unknowns.

When tens of millions of people start to take a drug – as is happening now – there could be some effects that we can't see coming. Gregg Stanwood is a developmental neuropharmacologist and neuroscientist at the College of Medicine at Florida State University, who has been researching GLP-1 agonists for years. He said he is broadly optimistic about these drugs – he's thinking of starting to take them himself, in fact. But he had a worry. He said he was fairly sure that in the short to medium term, if the drugs had a 'catastrophic' effect, 'we would know by now', because of all the diabetics using them. But if it is 'something slow and gradual, and takes a long time to present', then we might not know – and we won't know for years.

He gave me an analogy. 'I want to be clear – I am not suggesting that these drugs are going to work in this way,' he said, but a comparison helps to explain his point. 'Antipsychotics were first introduced in the 1950s, and have been used for a long time, relatively safely.' But one thing emerged over the very long term that nobody could have anticipated at the start.

It turns out that for people who have been taking them for decades, when they become elderly, it 'significantly increases the likelihood that they're going to develop at least dementia, if not full-blown Alzheimer's disease. It also greatly increases the likelihood they're going to have a falling incident and break a hip. But it took decades to get that [knowledge], because we needed a population that was on antipsychotics for a prolonged period of time and were ageing.' The drugs looked relatively safe for a very long time – until way down the line, when this effect finally showed up.

~

I put all my concerns about the potential risks to the companies who make these drugs, to see what they had to say. Novo Nordisk – who make Ozempic and Wegovy – sent a detailed response, which you can read in full in the endnotes. They said that these drugs are only available on prescription from a doctor or other healthcare professional, and they should only be taken under their supervision and in line with medical advice. Novo Nordisk stressed that they take patient safety very seriously and 'continuously monitor the safety profile of our medicines.' They reiterated the point Daniel Drucker had made to me: that these drugs have been studied in extensive clinical trials and used to treat diabetes for more than fifteen years and to treat obesity for eight years. By now, they said, these drugs have cumulatively 'had over 12 million patient years of exposure.'

They declined to comment specifically on some of the risks I asked about, like malnutrition or the loss of pleasure in food that some people taking the drugs are reporting.

On some of my other concerns, they did respond. When it comes to thyroid cancer, they underscored that the European Medicines Agency has said there is no evidence for a link with GLP-1 agonists. (However, their own safety leaflet that comes with the drugs in the US tells people with a history of thyroid cancer not to use them.) On pancreatitis, they said that this is an officially listed adverse reaction, but that for their drugs these side effects were generally mild to moderate in severity and of short duration. They pointed me towards a 'reassuring' study, which found that over thirty-nine months, people taking semaglutide were no more likely to develop pancreatitis than people taking a placebo. When it comes to muscle mass, they said that they did not study this question in their clinical trials, but pointed me towards one small sub-study of 140 people, where the people in the experiment did lose muscle mass, but they lost more fat mass. They then said that anyone experiencing this or any other side effects should discuss it with their doctor.

Eli Lilly, who make Mounjaro, declined to comment on any of the concerns I put to them.

~

In the face of uncertainty, we all have a decision to make. Shauna told me: 'We don't know the long-term side effects' of these new weight-loss drugs, 'but we do know the long-term side effects of living with obesity'. You have to choose your risk.

But presented with this dilemma, I began to ask – isn't there a third option?

6

Why Don't You Diet and Exercise Instead?

The two biggest alternatives to weight-loss drugs – and why they have (mostly) failed

All along, as I was weighing the risks of taking these drugs against the risks of continuing to be obese, I couldn't shake off a nagging doubt that I was a fool for even asking these questions – because there was a better, and blatantly obvious, solution that I could choose instead. I had dinner with a friend one night, and as he shovelled some breaded chicken schnitzel into his mouth, he said to me: 'I don't get it. Why don't you lose weight the normal way? Why don't you go on a diet and exercise instead?'

He was only asking what I had been thinking at the back of my own mind. Why do you need these risky drugs? Why don't you just show some willpower instead?

As we have grown fatter over the past forty years, we have been sold three different tools for weight loss. The first two are offered to us explicitly, while the third is only offered implicitly. They are exercise, diet and stigma. The recipe for weight loss, we are taught, is simple: eat less, move more and feel bad about yourself if you don't.

Ever since I was in my late teens, I have diligently tried to follow this script, usually around once a year. It has followed a familiar drumbeat. I would eliminate some type of food – carbohydrates, say – and eat less, while also exercising more. It worked: I would lose weight. Then my feeling of hunger would rage back, and seem much stronger than it had before. I would feel exhausted, crack – and then feel ashamed. I would resolve that next time, my willpower would be stronger.

This desire for the perfect diet has lured me down some strange alleyways over the years. When I was twenty-six, a friend of mine came back from a weight-loss clinic in Austria shimmering with apparent good health. She explained that the Mayr Clinic near Klagenfurt specialised in 'intestinal cleansing therapy' – if you spent a week there, they would clear your system of the toxins that build up and make you crave unhealthy food. I decided to head there.

I was greeted at the entrance by a woman dressed in an elaborate nineteenth-century Austrian peasant costume, who gave me a broad Stepford smile. As she walked me in, she said: 'Up until his death at the age of ninety – when he was incredibly mentally alert and active – Dr Mayr outlined visionary theories about the intestines. How happy he would have been about the spread of his theories! How happy he would have been to see you here!' She indicated a portrait of Dr Mayr, looking severe, staring down at us all.

She took me through to the restaurant, where I was given a bowl with a tiny puddle of soup at the bottom, and a piece of stale bread. 'I hear this is our last meal for the whole first week!' the woman next to me said with a masochistic grin.

'Excuse me,' I said. 'Why is the bread stale?' 'This is a good question,' the hostess replied. 'It is stale because we want to teach you to chew. Nobody in the Western world knows how to chew. Dr Mayr showed this. Most people today swallow their food after giving it one or two chews, and it enters the intestines very hard. This puts stress on the gut. Here, you will learn to chew each mouthful of food forty times.' Forty? 'Yes. Do not swallow anything until it is a thin liquid pulp. And you must not speak to each other or read when you are eating. This is distracting and wrong. You will sit in silence. And chew.'

Shortly afterwards, I was led by this refugee from the set of *Heidi* to meet Herr Doktor. Tall, in his late thirties, and earnest, he looked at my tongue and my eyes with a torch and a concerned expression. He took me to a mirror. 'Please put out your tongue and tell me what colour it is,' he said.

'Pink,' I replied.

'No. Please look again.' I peered. It was true – there was a distinctly non-pink fuzz. 'Mr Hari, your tongue is grey with elements of yellow.' He paused, shook his head, and added: 'This is not good. And now look at your eyes. They too are yellow.' I looked carefully: this I couldn't accept. 'Yes, they are. Look. There is a yellow tinge in the corners. This is a sign of a stressed and unhappy liver.' He scribbled something on his pad and told me to lie down 'so I can get the feeling of your intestines'. I lay back on his table in my underwear. He kept muttering to himself. 'Ah, the lower intestine – it is obscured,' he said at one point. And then – triumphantly – 'There is much gas here.'

'I think, Mr Hari, we will put you on the T Diet,' he said. I assumed he had twenty-six plans, running from A to Z, and he had plucked a special one for me. 'What does this diet involve?'

I enquired. 'For breakfast, you will have tea. And for lunch, you will have tea. And for dinner, you will have tea – with a hint of honey.' 'Ah,' I said. 'And when will I eat?' He paused again. 'You will eat tea – as you like. But there is a strict limit on the honey.'

I wandered down to the lake and found an Austrian woman lying listlessly on a recliner. She told me she been on the tea diet for two weeks. 'How do you feel?' I asked. 'Terrible,' she replied. 'And there is an Irish gentleman on the tea diet over there who has begun to hallucinate.'

Several days passed in a blur like this, talking to disorientated and starving people, and feeling my stomach slowly digest itself. Soon, I had a brutal headache. When I asked for an aspirin, the Austrian peasant woman handed me a tube. 'Attach this to the tap in your bedroom and give yourself an enema,' she said. On the third day, I was led into the basement for a treatment. There were four people in the room who all had what seemed to be giant cotton strips jammed up their nostrils, with tears running down their cheeks. I was told that they were having a 'nasal treatment'. (For some reason, this sounds even more sinister in German.) As a different nineteenth-century Austrian peasant approached me with something to jam up my nose, I walked out.

On day four, I awoke at three in the morning, drooling after a dream where I had drowned inside a gigantic strawberry milkshake. In a frenzy, I gathered up the fluff underneath my bed, and seriously considered eating it. I scampered down to the kitchen determined to raid it, but it had been locked away like a supply of gold bullion: even with all my strength (or what remained of it), I could not break into the stock of stale rolls.

Enough. I demanded an appointment with the doctor and told him I could not take this any more. He stroked his facial hair and said, 'I think you are lacking in courage, Mr Hari.' 'No, I am lacking in food,' I replied. 'Very well. We will give you a meal.' A meal! I nearly kissed him. I went to the restaurant – and was given something that would barely constitute a snack in the outside world: a tiny chunk of pizza, about the size of an Oreo. At tables all around me, the blank-eyed people 'eating' tea with honey in it stared at me, their mouths watering. I felt like Jack Nicholson in *One Flew Over the Cuckoo's Nest*, and wondered if I should start an uprising. I ate the fragment of pizza, packed my belongings, and fled, flicking a V-sign at Dr Mayr's portrait on the way out. The woman in Austrian peasant costume who had greeted me on the first day waved me goodbye, her smile not cracking for a moment.

Yet even with a diet as mad as this, when I got home, I felt like a failure. Where, I wondered, was my willpower?

~

Since the late 1950s, scientists have been putting people on diets and tracking how many of them succeed over time at losing weight. The logic behind using diet as a tool for weight loss is blindingly obvious. As you go through your day, you take in calories through food and drink, and you burn calories by moving. If you take in more calories than you burn, you create a calorie surplus, and you gain weight. If you burn more calories than you consume, you create a calorie deficit, and you lose weight. There's very broad scientific agreement that these principles are true. To dispute them, you have to dispute the basic laws of physics. This is why, at first, diets almost always do work. If you run a calorie deficit, you really will lose weight for a while. In the Mayr Clinic, I lost half a stone. At any given time, around 17 per cent of us are on a diet, and most people have been on one at some point in their lifetimes, so you are likely to remember how this feels. You discipline yourself, you eat less, and you feel your body change.

But scientists who investigate how diets work over the longer term have persistently bumped into something odd.

Traci Mann is a professor of psychology at the University of Minnesota who has carried out some of the most detailed long-term analyses of the effects of diets. When I asked her for an interview, she suggested we meet up at Isles Bun, a famous bakery in Minneapolis. As soon as I walked through the door, the guy behind the counter asked if I had been there before, and when I said I hadn't, he gave me a free bun smothered in butter, cinnamon, sugar and frosting. I placed it politely on the table in front of me, and resolved not to eat it as I waited for Traci.

When she sat down and started sipping coffee, she told me she had become curious about the effects of dieting when she was a grad student at Stanford in the final days of the twentieth century. Dieting was everywhere and she wanted to see how well it worked, so when she became an assistant professor at the University of California, Los Angeles, she decided to carry out a systematic review of all the research into the phenomenon up to that point. She began by asking a specific question. We all know there's short-term benefits to diets, but how well do they work in the longer term? After two years of dieting, how much weight has the average person successfully kept off? She read through over 2,000 scientific studies, and noticed something peculiar. They were full of claims that diets are extremely successful at producing weight loss – but most of the studies stopped after three months. They acted as if you lose weight in those first few months and then you stay at that lower level for ever, with your problem solved. But was that true?

She could find only twenty-one studies that had followed dieters rigorously for two years, or, in a few cases, five years. So what did they discover? It turned out that two years after starting a diet and making a real effort to stick at it, you will – on average – weigh two pounds less than you did at the start. It's almost nothing. This means the vast majority of diets fail. Traci was baffled. 'It was like up is down, left is right, dogs were cats,' she told me. 'Everything I read was the exact opposite of everything I'd been told my whole life. It was showing diets don't work.' She has now been researching dieting for more than twenty years, and she keeps finding similar outcomes. 'It seems that they work for the initial weight loss, and then back on it comes.'

But how could this be? It's a scientific fact that if you burn more calories than you consume, you will lose weight. So what is getting in the way of that?

For me, this question also took a different form. If we all gained weight because we stopped eating like my Swiss ancestors, why doesn't eating like my Swiss ancestors now bring us back to looking like them?

It seemed to make no sense. But then I learned there is an answer, though it's a complicated one.

~

When I was researching my books on addiction and depression, I kept asking experts what caused these problems, and

I was introduced to a crucial part of the answer. It's there in all the textbooks, though it is rarely explained to the public. It is called the 'bio-psycho-social model'. This sounds technical, but it's actually simple, and it applies just as well to obesity. There are three types of cause of these problems. There's biological causes – things like your genes, or changes in your brain. There's psychological causes – things like stress, or childhood trauma. And there's social causes, stemming from the wider society – things like loneliness, or financial insecurity. They are all real, and they play out, to differing degrees, in anyone who has these problems. These different kinds of cause flow into your life and swirl together to create your addiction, or depression, or obesity, and it explains why we have become obese, and why diets mostly fail.

Let's start with the biology. As you gain weight, a series of transformations take place in your body and brain that make it very hard for you to ratchet back. Michael Lowe, the expert on hunger at Drexel University, explained to me that back in the 1960s and 70s, when he began his work, scientists believed that when you are born, you have a natural 'set point' that is innate to your brain and determines what weight you are going to be for the rest of your life. They thought it was 'very much like the set point we have for body temperature. When we're born, we have a built-in system that pre-sets our body temperature at 98 degrees, and we have all kinds of mechanisms to keep it there.' If you get too hot, you sweat to cool down. If you get too cold, you shiver, which raises your body temperature. Your brain and body act automatically to keep you at this set point, and it's very hard to get outside it.

Body weight, the scientists reckoned, was similar. Just as your body keeps you at a certain temperature, it keeps you at a certain weight that's built into your body from birth. If you start to go outside that innate range, it uses all sorts of mechanisms to pull you back to the weight you should be. If you get thinner than your set point, it will make you ragingly hungry. If you get fatter than your set point, it will make you feel sick to put you off food. But 'then we experienced the obesity epidemic. Well, the obesity epidemic is totally inconsistent with the notion of a set point, because our average weights are going up and up.'

They realised they had to adjust this theory – but how? After decades of studying the evidence, Michael was convinced that 'we do have a set point – but it is acquired, not preset'. As you gain weight, your biological set point – the weight your brain tries to keep your body at – rises and rises. Imagine if, every time it got hotter, your body's temperature set point adjusted upwards. You went to the Sahara Desert, and your body tried to keep you – for ever after – at the clammier, hotter levels you experienced there. Michael came to believe that something like this really does happen with your weight. 'If somebody gains thirty pounds over, say, five years, and they stay there for several months, the body now biologically treats that thirty-pound extra weight as its new defensible set point.' It takes your new higher weight as the natural one, and 'it does not react well if you try to dislodge your weight from that'.

So if you gain weight and then try to cut back, all sorts of biological mechanisms – the equivalent of sweating and shivering when the temperature changes – start to kick in. Your metabolism slows down, and you burn calories more slowly. But Traci, the expert on diet failure, added: 'It's not just metabolism. Your hormone levels change. You're more likely to be hungry and less likely to be full. There's all kinds of attentional changes so you're more likely to notice food … Once you notice food, it's hard to not pay attention to it any more. You just become pre-occupied with thoughts of food.' Your body releases less energy, so you don't want to move as much. Your brain will send signals to make you crave more fatty and sugary foods.

That, I realised, is what happened to me on every diet I ever went on. It's what was happening to me in the Mayr Clinic by day four, as the dreams of strawberry milkshake came to me in the night.

Why would our brains do this to us? It is, Michael says, for reasons deep in our evolution as a species. It's 'a biological adaptation. Remember: the body's tendency to do this – over the millions of years that we evolved – was a brilliant survival strategy. The problem for millions of years wasn't how to avoid eating too much. It was to make sure we constantly had enough to eat.' Our ancestors, when it came to food, faced one big problem: famine. You were quite likely, at some point in your life, to experience your food supply drying up or disappearing altogether. To protect against this, as soon you gained some fat, your body thought: Good, let's keep this, because when the next famine comes, we can burn through this fat store and survive. The more fat stores, the better, because at the end of a famine, the person who was fattest at the start will be the last man standing. This is why our bodies evolved to see every gain in weight as a new 'acquired set point', he says – one it should fight to maintain. It's why we have an innate 'bodily tendency to hold on to what we have'.

In the circumstances where we evolved, this was a very good system. It kept us alive. But in the circumstances where we now live, it's killing lots of us. Today, the problem we face isn't famine, it's having too much food. 'Evolution could never have anticipated that we would have an abundance of energy [sources] all the time,' Michael explained. 'The system was designed for one environment that took millions of years to create, and now it's trying to cope with a radically different environment.'

This is why, when we try to lose weight, 'we are prevented from maintaining those weight losses by the reactions in our body'. It sees holding on to more fat as good, and losing fat as bad – and it will try to keep you at your fattest. When Robert De Niro gained weight for the movie *Raging Bull*, he was stunned by how hard it was to lose it: he said it was like his body was fighting to stay at the higher level. He was right. 'Of course, that's really bad news for individuals with obesity,' Michael said, 'because they're fighting their biology, and their biology is, in effect, 24/7.' This is 'a perfect storm not only for weight gain, but for weight regain after weight loss'.

Many scientists explained this theory to me, in urgent tones. Dr Giles Yeo, the researcher at Cambridge University, said: 'Your brain hates it when you lose weight. It will drag you kicking and screaming back up to where you were ... I'm a 75-kilogram human being. Imagine if I had a twin who was 85 kilos, and he lost ten kilos to become my weight. Because my now 75-kilo twin has lost weight, he will have to eat less than me in order to maintain exactly the same weight, because his brain is thinking "I have lost ten kilos. I've lowered my metabolism. I'm going to now keep the metabolism low, until you get back up to where you were before."' It was put to me even more bluntly by Jerold Mande, the professor of nutrition at Harvard. 'The body always fights back,' he said. 'We have billions of years of evolution to make sure that weight gets back within five years.'

That's the biological part of why it's so hard to lose weight and so easy to regain it. I learned a lot about the psychological factors for a chapter that you'll come to a little later.

Then there's the environmental component. When you go on a diet, you try, as an individual, to lose weight – but, as Giles Yeo put it, 'you're trying to change your diet in the food environment we're already living in.' You can't isolate yourself from it. We all live in an environment where shitty food is cheap, constantly promoted to us and pushed in our faces, while healthy food is expensive, unpromoted and harder to get. In fact, many people live in 'food deserts', places where it is impossible to buy fresh food at affordable prices. Michael Lowe calls this kind of environment 'obesogenic' – we live in a society that makes it easy to become obese, and hard to go back. In fact, he told me, 'we have an environment that is about as obesogenic as man could design.'

So when you try to change as an individual, you are doing it in an obesogenic environment that has not changed – and is pushing you to go back to eating the way you did before. We mostly fail, Michael said, because 'the problem we are dealing with is essentially bigger than us.'

This was depressing. It means that diets fail most of the time because we are sabotaged by our biology and our environment.

Some people can – through some combination of luck, supportive family, helpful genes, and/or staggering willpower – lose weight and keep it off. It's also true that some people manage to climb Mount Everest without extra oxygen, and some people win big on the roulette wheels in Vegas. But the odds are rigged against you.

When I saw weight in this context, I realised that my fixation on willpower – one day I'll have enough! – had been too simplistic. Willpower is real. But out of all the biological, psychological and social causes, it is just one sliver of one of those sets of causes. To say it's irrelevant and plays no role in controlling weight is wrong; but to say it's everything – or even most of the picture – is equally wrong. Willpower is one fragile factor in a big and complicated picture. It is like an umbrella in a nasty storm. It will provide you with some protection. For a few people, it will get them to their destination. But for most of us, it will be broken by bigger forces.

~

Sitting in the Minneapolis bakery, Traci almost took the words out of my mouth when she said: 'People often say, "Well, if what you're saying about dieting is true, how come Joe X in my social group has lost weight and kept it off?" The answer is – it's not impossible. I am talking about the general pattern. The most likely pattern.' In most areas of science, she said, 'there's usually outliers', but dieting is the only area where the scientists involved become 'obsessed with the minority result' and present it as if it's typical. Most diet researchers, in her experience, 'just couldn't get over their focus on what a small fraction of their patients achieved. You don't see that in any other type of study. [Normally] we look at what happens on average, and the variability around that, but we don't harp on the tiny subset of people who do something very different than the rest. Obviously it's possible – if you starve someone, they become emaciated, right?' But in the environment where we live, with the biology we have, it's ferociously hard. Most people will fail. And it's not, she stressed, their fault.

As she was speaking, almost absent-mindedly, I found myself eating the sugar-soaked cinnamon bun they gave me for free. She leaned in to my recorder, and said: 'Let the record show he is eating the frosting with his finger.'

~

Some scientists are a little more optimistic about diets than Traci, but the margin of hope is surprisingly small. In 2001, a team at the University of Kentucky analysed all the best scientific studies of structured weight-loss programmes in the US, and found that five years after taking part, the average person was less overweight by a statistically significant amount: 6.6 pounds, or around 3 per cent of their body weight. It's not nothing – but it's not much. Another team at Brown Medical School in Rhode Island surveyed the limited evidence we have, including a study that tracked over time 4,000 people who have successfully lost a lot of weight. They found that roughly 20 per cent of people are successful with diets, if you define success as losing at least 10 per cent of your body weight, and maintaining that loss for at least a year. This isn't a picture of total hopelessness. One in five people being able to improve their health through diet, even a little, is valuable. But it's not a lot.

~

I also wanted to know: what about the other tool we are sold as The Answer – exercise? To understand the role it can play in promoting weight loss, I went to see for myself a curious experiment. For a moment, you might wonder why I am telling you this story – but stick with me. The experiment began as a programme to stop kids smoking, boozing and taking drugs – but it turned into the most successful programme anywhere in the world at promoting exercise in young people.

In 1950, in a remote fishing village on the west coast of Iceland, a six-year-old boy named Thorolfur Thorlindsson was afraid. He was sitting with his grandfather in the basement of his house, as the old man smelted together some wires to fix the engine on his fishing boat. Suddenly, a spark from his welding equipment made some papers on the floor nearby burst into flames. Thorolfur panicked and ran away. His grandfather calmly put out the fire, and then called Thorolfur back, and sat the little boy down. 'Were you scared?' he asked. Thorolfur didn't answer. 'Courage is just a matter of habit,' the old man explained. 'So you can right now start to practise being scared, or you can practise being brave.'

His grandfather had learned to be brave the hard way. He had to take his fishing boat out in all sorts of weather, on a part of the coast that is both battered by the westerly winds and often smothered by fog. He told Thorolfur: 'If you're out there on the sea, nobody's going to help you. You have to trust in yourself. You have to relax. You have to concentrate. Part of the skill of dealing with bad weather on a small boat is concentrating. You have to focus on every wave. If you lose your focus, you're probably gone.' One time in December, he was way out at sea when a blizzard struck. There were only two of them on the boat, alone. Their instinct was to row frantically against the wind to try to get back to shore, but their better judgement told them it was impossible, and if they tried, they would drown. So they had to do something risky – steer to one side, and hope that even in that white snowy miasma, they could judge it precisely so the boat would hit the south corner of the fjord. He knew that if they missed it, they would be carried far out to sea, and die. He said: 'Always, under pressure, stay cool.'

Forty years later, Thorolfur faced a crisis of his own, and he thought of his grandfather's words. Iceland had been gradually moving away from being a fishing and farming country, and in this transition, a lot of people became disorientated. Young Icelandic people in particular seemed to be in trouble. In villages and towns across the country, on the long summer nights, teenagers would gather in crowds of hundreds, and get drunk or high. Raucous fights would break out. Older people became afraid to go out. At the same time, younger people were moving away from the healthier diet of their ancestors, towards a more Western diet – and, as in every country where this change happens, obesity was beginning to rise.

As a sociologist, Thorolfur was shocked by the evidence about how widespread these problems were for Iceland's young people. As Inga Dora Sigfusdottir, who worked with him as a researcher, told me: 'Icelandic adolescents were much more likely to binge-drink than kids in other parts of Europe … In 1998, 42 per cent of fifteen-year-old kids had become drunk in the past thirty days. Twenty per cent were daily smokers. Seventeen per cent had tried hashish.' These large crowds of drunk and drugged kids shocked the country. A woman named Sunna, who was one of those troubled youths, told me: 'I think a lot of us were lost. Lost, and looking for a way in life … I just didn't care. I didn't care about myself. I didn't have a lot of esteem for myself. I had a lot of anger, and didn't know how to let that out.'

At first, Icelanders thought the solution was obvious. Schools taught kids to Just Say No – to drugs, and to unhealthy food.

They tried to terrify the kids with horror stories about where this behaviour would take them and their health. Thorolfur thought this was all wrong.

So he proposed to solve the problem in a very different way. He set up a government-backed initiative called Youth in Iceland, which was designed to help kids experience 'natural highs'. When you accomplish something – especially something physical – you get a rush of endorphins and satisfaction that matches a drug high. To achieve this, the initiative created a huge network of youth and sports clubs across the country. Every child was given a voucher, twice a year, by the government, to pay for access to something physically active and endorphin-pumping that they wanted to do – sport, or dance, or music.

I went to see one of these centres in the neighbourhood of Throttur in Reykjavik. I was shown around by Gudberg Jonsson, who runs part of the programme. The first thing I saw was a football pitch, lit up by floodlights, with girls playing on it. 'In this club now, we have eleven sports,' he said, and started to list them off: 'taekwondo, track and field, Olympic lifting, powerlifting, skiing, swimming, gymnastics ...' We stepped into one of the first buildings, which looked more like an Olympic Village than a youth centre. We walked from the basketball pitch to the ice-skating rink, past a room where teenage boys were trampolining, doing triple flips in the air, and another room where I saw what looked like a massive flash-mob, with kids of all different ages teaching each other a synchronised dance.

'The lights are on until at least ten o'clock in all these buildings,' every day of the week, he told me. It's voluntary, but almost all Icelandic kids take part. 'All their friends are doing something, so you'll find something that will be of interest to you.' Now, as a result of this programme, virtually every Icelandic child and teen takes part in many hours of vigorous exercise every week. The kids I spoke to loved the programme and enjoyed the exercise it offered – including the kids who were on the larger side, who in the US and Britain would (like I did at their age) have scorned this sort of thing.

The programme has been stunningly successful. At the start, 42 per cent of kids were getting drunk regularly. Today, it's 8 per cent. Rates of teenage smoking and drug use also fell dramatically. They went from having some of the highest rates of alcohol, drug and tobacco use in Europe, to some of the lowest.

And obesity among young people? At the same time as all these other amazing outcomes, youth obesity continued to rise dramatically. Despite having the most successful exercise programme in Europe, Icelandic kids are among the fattest on the continent.

How can this be? It seemed baffling. But then I learned that it fits with a much wider body of evidence about exercise. For example, a team of scientists at Arizona State University got eighty-one women to walk on a treadmill for half an hour, three times a week, for three months, and they tracked what happened to the women's weight. Incredibly, fifty-five of them put on weight. Two-thirds of them gained fat mass. The evidence is clear that exercise rarely causes sustained weight loss. A different study found that only 2 per cent of people who lost 2.2 stone or more, and kept it off for twelve months, achieved it solely by exercising.

The scientists who have studied these apparently perverse findings say there are a few reasons for them. The first is that in the environment we live in, the small number of calories you burn by increasing exercise are quickly swamped by the ongoing rise in calories that come in through food. Tim Spector, who has studied so many aspects of obesity, told me bluntly: 'You can't run off a bad diet.' We hugely overestimate how many calories are burned by exercise, and what we can eat to treat ourselves afterwards. If you eat a large Big Mac meal, you'd have to run for roughly two hours without a break to burn off those calories. Even for a single Snickers bar, you'd need to run intensely for around twenty minutes. In Iceland, over the period the Youth in Iceland programme was rolled out, the kids exercised far more – but at the same time, their eating habits were much worse. The bad diet trumped the good exercise.

Does this mean we should just give up on exercise then? Everyone I spoke to said that was a terrible idea, and that exercise massively boosts your health and quality of life, irrespective of whether it triggers weight loss. If you don't exercise enough, you are more likely to develop over forty chronic diseases, ranging broadly from diabetes to colon cancer. Tim Spector said: 'It's really important for preventing many diseases, for your mental health, for anti-ageing, anti-dementia, [preventing] cancers and heart diseases. You name it.' If you exercise for 270 hours a year, you'll add, on average, three years to your life.

Exercise works unbelievably well at preventing all sorts of problems, from heart attacks and strokes to an early death. What it doesn't work well at is – alas – producing weight loss.

~

After studying all this, I kept thinking back to the shame I felt when I cracked and gave up on the diets and exercise programmes

I had tried. What has it done to us psychologically, to become fatter, and to be insistently offered a solution that in fact mostly fails? I discussed this with lots of people, including a woman named Julie who approached me after reading online that I was writing about Ozempic. She told me that she has been fighting against her body weight her whole adult life. 'I've beaten myself up for years for not having enough willpower – for being lazy, even though I exercise every day and even though I try to eat healthily. I failed time and time again, giving in to cravings that were seemingly beyond my control.' She believed 'weight is all about diet and exercise and willpower, and obesity is a choice. All of it is a choice. And I was a failure about it, over and over again … I realised how closely tied my depression was to my failures trying to make myself healthy. It was – try, fail, berate myself, try, fail, berate myself. Try and fail, hate myself.'

~

And yet, even after I absorbed all of this, I found it very hard to give up on believing in these two solutions. The idea that one day I would sustainably lose weight by eating better and exercising was a core part of how I thought about my future, and it had been since I was a teenager. As I learned the evidence that they rarely work, it felt like the lights were fading on a stage, and the play I was sure I was going to star in one day was disappearing before my eyes.

The truth is that in the environment that has been created in the past forty years, it is extraordinarily hard to lose weight and keep it off. This, it seemed to me, was one of the biggest arguments for these drugs. We are trapped, and this is the trapdoor.

When I injected myself with Ozempic for the fifth month in a row, I thought of all the diets I had tried over the years, all the times I had tried to cut out carbs, or sugar. I pictured those poor starving people at the Mayr Clinic, weird objects rammed up their noses, tears streaming down their faces, seeking any solution, no matter how wild.

I wondered if all those diets had been a sad joke all along, and this was my only option now.

7

The Brain Breakthrough

Good news for addiction, bad news for depression?

Six months after I started taking Ozempic, I noticed something. Every morning, when I woke up, I experienced two sensations at the same time. I felt that my body was shrinking. I could put my hands on my stomach and feel that where I had been pot-bellied, I was now lean. I felt fitter, and better-looking, and more confident. But I also felt something else. My mood was strangely muted. I didn't feel as excited for the day ahead as I normally do. I felt a little listless. I don't want to overstate this – I wasn't depressed. I was often emotionally dulled.

It certainly wasn't an all-consuming feeling. I had moments of feeling really happy. I was getting more attention from men, and people kept complimenting me on the change in my appearance. But on the whole, I felt that my mood was slightly lower than it had been before I started taking these drugs, and I was puzzled. Why would I feel like this, when I was getting what I wanted? It's possible it was just a coincidence, and other things in my life unrelated to the drugs were bringing me down. But, I wondered, was Ozempic having a negative effect on my state of mind?

As I investigated this, it led me into a deeper set of topics related to these drugs. There are two schools of thought that could explain this reaction to these drugs – one biological and one psychological. Perhaps these drugs were primarily affecting my biology – particularly my brain – in ways that made me feel worse. Or perhaps they were mostly affecting my psychology.

I looked at the brain effects first. To get to their potential effects on depression, I had to first understand the debate about what they are doing to our brains more generally – and, intriguingly, what that might mean for people with addiction problems.

~

When these drugs were first being discovered, it seemed that the reason why they worked was simple. As I explained in chapter one, they are an artificial copy of a gut hormone – GLP-1 – that tells you when you're full. The real hormone lasts for a few minutes and then vanishes; the replica lingers for a whole week. They work primarily in your gut and on your gut, boosting fullness and slowing digestion. That's their secret.

But then there was an unexpected breakthrough. GLP-1 was discovered in the first place because, in the early 1980s, scientists had new techniques that made it possible to study the inner workings of human cells in a way that hadn't been possible before. Not long after, something similar happened with the brain: there were huge advances in how scientists could see into it, and they started to discover all sorts of things that nobody had seen coming. One of them related to GLP-1. Using these new methods, a team at Hammersmith Hospital in London stumbled on an unexpected fact. Studying rats, they found that there are receptors for GLP-1 – areas of the body particularly sensitive to it – far from the gut. It turned out that they actually have receptors for GLP-1 in their brains. It seemed peculiar, and led to the obvious question: is this also true of humans? It turned out it was. Then it was discovered that all humans actually *make* GLP-1 in their brains. It was a bombshell. We don't just process and make this hormone in our guts. We process and make it in our brains.

This led to more questions. When you inject people with a GLP-1 agonist like semaglutide – which is marketed as Ozempic and Wegovy – where does the effect actually play out? Robert Kushner, who had played a key role in developing Wegovy, told me: 'If you do animal studies and you tag the compound' and then 'you look at where it goes in a rodent's brain, it's everywhere. It's deep in the brain – in the appetite centre, in the reward centres and the homeostatic centres.' Dr Clemence Blouet, who is researching this question at Cambridge University, agreed, saying the receptors for these drugs are 'in lots of different areas … It's everywhere'.

So scientists began to ask: when you take these drugs, is it possible that the reduction in appetite isn't driven primarily by changing the chemicals in your gut, but by changing your brain?

At first glance, this might sound like a technical question. You could say: Who cares, so long as it works? But in fact, this reframing of how GLP-1 agonists work made scientists wonder if there was a possible set of uses for these drugs that nobody had asked yet. If it works on your brain, might the drug also be able to shape more than just the way you eat? As they dug further, they started to ask an extraordinary question. Had they, in fact, discovered a drug that boosts self-control across the board? If they had, might it be used to treat addiction?

At the same time, some of them worried that the fact that the drug works on the brain also opened up a new set of risks. If it's changing your brain for the better, could it also potentially change it for the worse? What kind of harm could the drugs be doing?

This change of focus – from the gut, to the brain – seemed like it could radically reframe how we think about these drugs. Of all the areas of science that I learned about for this book, this was both the most complex, and the one where scientists are most uncertain. There's a huge amount we don't know, and the scientists involved all counsel that we need to approach this topic with a heavy dollop of humility. As I read their work and talked it over with them, I felt like I was staring at a fuzzy picture that was only very slowly coming into shape. We can only glimpse broad contours of the potential positive and negative effects of these drugs on the brain for now – and it's important to know going in that some of what we think we can see might turn out to be an illusion. Clemence said: 'Some people say the brain is the most complex object in the universe,' so it's hardly surprising that when it comes to these drugs, 'we're still trying to understand how everything works'.

~

In 2013, in a lab in Pennsylvania, a young neuroscientist named Diana Williams did something nobody had ever done before. She injected GLP-1 directly into the part of a rat's brain known as the nucleus accumbens. This is a key part of what scientists call 'the reward centres'. Paul Kenny, who carried out the Cheesecake Park experiment, explained to me what they are. 'The reward centres are there to keep you alive … If you're hungry and you eat food, the reason the food feels pleasurable is because you engage those pleasure centres in your brain.' The same goes for when you have sex, or connect with other people, or listen to great music – all of these activities make your reward centres hum. 'The role of those centres is to encourage you to approach, obtain and consume factors that are required for life and its propagation.' This is 'absolutely crucial', because 'if you don't experience pleasure from the things that are important for sustaining, maintaining and propagating life, there's a very good chance that you won't engage in those types of behaviours.'

Diana discovered that the rats who'd had GLP-1 jabbed into their nucleus accumbens ate significantly less. Up to that point, scientists had tried injecting GLP-1 into other parts of rats' brains, but – she told me – 'these reward-related brain areas had been, up to this point ignored.' Now she began to wonder: was the key to changing somebody's desire for food, in fact, to change how rewarding they find it?

Were the reward centres the key to the positive effects of these drugs? Or was something else going on?

~

When Heath Schmidt heard about the results of the early experiments to inject GLP-1 agonists directly into rodents' brains, his spider-sense began to tingle. He is the director of the Lab of Neuropsychopharmacology at the University of Pennsylvania, and has been studying addiction for his entire career. He told me he was particularly struck by one finding. If a GLP-1 agonist is jabbed into a rat's brain, it will massively cut back on its consumption of junk food – but it will eat just as much of the normal, healthy rat chow. 'So you can think of it as – we're sitting here and we have a choice between a salad and a Happy Meal from McDonald's. Most of the time, we're going for the Happy Meal. But if you squirt this drug into the [area of the brain known as the] VTA [which is also part of the reward system], we're going to reduce our desire to eat the Happy Meal, but leave our eating of the salad intact.'

This is really unusual and significant, he said, for one key reason. In the past, scientists had tried designing drugs to reduce addictive behaviours, but they kept bumping into a problem. They could find drugs that dampened addiction, but the drugs also dampened 'natural rewarding behaviours, like feeding and sex and social interactions'. They worked by dialling down your entire reward system, so if you took them, you lost your interest in cocaine, but you also lost your interest in life and all of its pleasures. That's not much use. 'The reality is that we're talking about the same circuits in the brain – so when you start mucking about with those circuits, you're going to affect all of those behaviours.' Until, he says, you get to these new weight-loss drugs. In the animal studies, they seemed at first glance to have some kind of 'selectivity' – to be able to distinguish between life-denying behaviours and life-enhancing behaviours, between Big Macs and salads.

It was, he said, 'a light-bulb moment – in the sense that this could be a really novel direction to go in that nobody's really thought about before'.

With this thought in mind, teams of scientists all over the world started to ask: could semaglutide be used to cut the use of drugs, from nicotine and alcohol, to heroin and cocaine, by people who've become addicted to them?

I spoke with several of the teams who have been investigating this. At the University of Gothenberg in Sweden, Elisabet Jerlhag, a professor of pharmacology, told me she had been intrigued for a long time by a curious fact. The brains of people addicted to cocaine look remarkably similar to the brains of people who are obese, or engage in binge-eating. Given the biological similarities of the problems, if there's a drug that works for one of these sets of compulsive behaviours, there's some chance it will work for the others too.

So she embarked on a series of experiments to find out. Her team took a group of rats and put them in a cage. As the rats got settled in, they discovered they had two water bottles – one filled with water, and the other with alcohol.

They quickly got drunk. When this happened, 'they wobble around, like humans'. At the end of every day, Elisabet would replenish the alcohol, and the rats would dash to it. She would hear them excitedly supping at the bottles. 'You can see they really enjoy and want to drink the alcohol.' Then, once the rat cage had become like a dive bar in North Las Vegas, they stepped in and staged an intervention. They injected the skin under the rats' necks with GLP-1 agonists, and then waited to see what would happen.

After being given the medication, the rats drank much less booze. The alcohol intake 'actually reduced by 60 per cent in some of these studies', Elisabet noted. 'So it's a quite dramatic effect.' The effect was most pronounced in the rats that consumed the most – the rough rat equivalents to alcoholics.

So Elisabet and her colleagues had discovered that GLP-1 drugs could reduce the total amount of alcohol that rats consumed. Next they wanted to explore something deeper: how they made the rats *feel* about alcohol. This is tricky: rats don't respond to interview questions. So they tried several more subtle experiments to tease this out.

Firstly, they designed a new cage. A rat is dropped into it, and he finds those bottles again – one with water, one with booze. But this time, the alcohol bottle works differently. There is a little lever at its base, and to get the booze, he needs to pump the lever with his paw. Initially, he only has to push the lever a few times, and the booze squirts out deliciously into his mouth. But after a few weeks, the scientists made it harder. To get it, the rat needs to work the lever ten times, twenty times, or more. This was a way of measuring how much the rat really wants the alcohol. If he's not very bothered about the booze, he'll give up early, while a rat that's motivated will pump and pump frantically to get his fix.

Elisabet discovered that if you inject a rat with a GLP-1 agonist, it will give up much sooner. The drug made them less excited by alcohol. It showed, she said, this 'GLP-1 receptor agonist reduces the reward of alcohol'.

This led them to another way of exploring the rats' feelings. When humans or rats drink alcohol, they often experience a rush of dopamine – the pleasure chemical. So they tested the brains of rats before and after being given a GLP-1 agonist. After the injection, they got less of a dopamine rush from booze. It really was changing the reward systems of their brains. It was making alcohol less fun.

If you consume alcohol heavily for a while, when you stop, you'll experience withdrawal effects, like sweating, tremors and being sick. It turns out this is true of rats too. Elisabet told me that if 'you inject them with alcohol for a long time and then you stop injecting, you can see that they have anxiety-like behaviours. They shiver.' But when she injected these withdrawal-stricken rats with GLP-1 agonists, she discovered that their symptoms significantly reduced. They felt the pain of losing alcohol much less keenly.

Finally, Elisabet and her team discovered that GLP-1 agonists had a positive effect in preventing another negative effect of addiction: relapse. They would give the rats alcohol for ten or twelve weeks, then take it away for two weeks, then reintroduce it. Normally, she said, 'when they get the alcohol back, they drink a lot' – more, in fact, than they were drinking before it was taken away. 'That's why it's called relapse drinking. That's exactly what you see in humans also. If you have a patient and they stop drinking alcohol, they have these abstinence symptoms, then they have a lot of craving and that makes them want to drink again, and when they start drinking, they drink more than they did before.' But when she gave the rats GLP-1 agonists, they were less likely to relapse.

I asked Elisabet why the drug has these effects. 'That's not completely known yet,' she said. She is confident one reason is that 'you block the reward from alcohol … They experience less reward, and that's why you don't want to continue drinking alcohol.'

But some scientists wondered if there could be something much more basic at work. Heath Schmidt told me that GLP-1 drugs reduce your desire for calories, and when you drink alcohol, 'you have something with caloric content that's filling up your stomach'. Could all this just be an effect of having less desire for calories?

There was a way to find out. Several scientists began to investigate if taking semaglutide could reduce the use of drugs that contain no calories. A team led by Patricia Grigson, the chair of the Department of Neural and Behavioral Sciences at Penn State University, explored whether giving GLP-1 agonists to rats cut their use of heroin or fentanyl. She discovered that it does, to a remarkable extent. She told me: 'It reduces their cue-induced seeking behaviours' – how much they try to get the drug – 'at least in half.' This shows GLP-1 agonists are 'very protective' in reducing excessive use. A team at Florida State University, involving Gregg Stanwood, did something similar: giving cocaine to mice. They found that GLP-1 agonists reduced the desire of rodents for coke by roughly 50 per cent. When he saw the results, Gregg said: 'Oh, this is damn cool. This is something that could really help people if we're able to get it out there.'

Many scientists who looked at these experiments were startled by one thing in particular: GLP-1 agonists didn't just reduce the desire for one drug, but it seemed for all drugs. Christian Hendershot, an associate professor of clinical psychology at the University of North Carolina, said: 'One of the compelling findings off the bat was that GLP-1 receptor agonists appeared to affect drug intake across different drug classes. When you look at all these different drugs – alcohol, nicotine, psychostimulants, even opioids – in almost all the studies, you see some kind of significant effect of the GLP-1 on drug intake. It's not very often that you would see a drug have widespread effects on addictive behaviours.' Obviously, he said, 'this could be extremely valuable if it turns out the drug does concurrently reduce – for example – drinking and smoking, two of the major sources of disease burden.'

As he said this, I asked myself – what if the idea that these are weight-loss drugs is kind of a mischaracterisation? What if they don't work primarily on your weight, but instead work primarily on your relationship with rewards – and reduce your cravings for things that can be bad for you across the board?

~

When Ozempic took off stratospherically in 2023, a lot of people taking it for weight loss started to notice something unexpected. I spoke with Tracey, a Canadian mental health worker in her mid-fifties, who developed a series of addictions after a marriage break-up. She would compulsively shop online, soothing herself by buying huge amounts of clothes she would never wear and books she would never read, feeling a rush every time she clicked the 'purchase' button. She was squandering the equivalent of a typical mortgage payment every month on her shopping addiction. She would compulsively binge on a lot of sweet foods, followed by a lot of savoury foods. And she started compulsively picking at her skin, tearing off tiny chunks. In combination, these addictive behaviours were 'definitely veering towards out of control'.

Her doctor prescribed Ozempic for weight loss, and around a month in, she noticed something. 'I don't have any cravings,' she told me. She had stopped compulsively shopping, binge-eating and picking at her skin. 'I don't have any desire to do it. There's no compulsion. It's like there was a need before – that's how I see addiction: as a visceral need to do this thing. Then it's just not there. My impulsivity has really decreased, which is really amazing.'

In North Carolina, Christian Hendershot was bombarded by doctors telling him that their patients, after a few months on the drug, were saying 'I don't feel like drinking any more

... I don't feel like smoking any more.' Lots of people started to offer anecdotal accounts of how the drug had led them to give up all sorts of compulsive behaviours, from gambling to pornography. He said: 'It's interesting because these are things we don't hear when we put people on the medications that are designed for addiction ... This stands out.' In London, the doctor Max Pemberton said: 'It was so noticeable that several of my friends who have a problem with alcohol ... experienced a revelation' after they started to take Ozempic. They said: ' "Oh my God, I can't believe that I'm now not drinking. Weeks have gone past, and I have no desire to drink." It felt to me that there's very much a neurological element to it.'

The scientists who had been investigating the effects of these drugs on animals were fascinated that the effects seemed, at first glance, to be translating to humans. Elisabet Jerlhag, who had shown how it worked on rats, said: 'I got very happy, because that's the hypothesis we have had for so many years ... It was confirming what we saw in our preclinical studies.' Patricia Grigson, who had shown the reduction in heroin use in rats, said: 'I'm not surprised, because of what we're seeing in the laboratory, but I'm amazed.'

Many scientists across the world are now giving GLP-1 agonists to people with addiction problems in clinical trials, and the results will come in gradually. We shouldn't be overly optimistic. Gregg Stanwood said: 'One of the issues we have in neuroscience is we get lots of quality leads in animals that don't translate well to people. Part of that might be differences in brain biology, but a lot of it at the end of the day is the complexity of the human condition that we simply can't model well in mice or any animal model. So I always want to be cautious.'

As I write this, we only have very provisional results for people, and they're something of a mixed bag. So far, it looks like GLP-1 agonists do reduce smoking – but only if you combine them with a nicotine patch. They do reduce alcohol use – but only in overweight people who had an alcohol problem in the first place. In a cocaine study, it didn't reduce use – but it made people a little less sensitive to triggers that would normally make them want to use.

These are all very small early studies, and we'll know a lot more in a few years. Heath Schmidt, who also conducted some of the key research, counselled: 'I want to be a cheerleader for clinical trials of these drugs, because I definitely think that there's enough data out there now to support them. But I also don't want to give people the false hope that these are going to be miracle drugs for all individuals with substance-use disorders. We just don't know at this point.'

~

Most people taking these drugs say that it changes how they think, and seems to have a profound effect on their brains. They find that the foods they have craved, and obsessed over, suddenly seem far less rewarding. The 'food chatter' that dominated their thinking dies down. To many of them, it feels much more like an effect in their skulls than on their guts.

But if the positive effects of the drug come in part from dampening the reward centres of the brain, this begs the obvious question: what are the downsides to doing that? Exploring this question led me to the eleventh potential risk associated with these drugs.

We know that other drugs interfering with the reward system of the brain have sometimes had very unpredictable results. For example, if you have Parkinson's disease, the dopamine neurons in your brain begin to deteriorate, so you might well be given a drug like L-Dopa to treat it. Wayne Hall, an emeritus professor of public health policy at the University of Queensland in Australia, told me that these drugs 'bump up dopamine levels in the brain', and it works – your Parkinson's symptoms become less pronounced. But after a few years, doctors started to notice it also occasionally produced a disturbing effect. Now that these patients had supercharged reward systems, they sometimes acted wildly out of character. They would rush out and gamble all their life savings. Men in their seventies who've been faithful to their wives all their married lives would suddenly start hitting on twenty-year-olds. The drugs 'turbo-charge the reward system, and produce this sort of compulsive behaviour'.

If that's what happens when you dramatically dial up your brain's reward system, what would be the result of potentially dialling down your brain's reward system? How selective can these drugs really be in distinguishing between different behaviours?

All the scientists I discussed this with proceeded cautiously, and stressed – again – that there's a lot we don't know about it. I am going to quote a lot of people here, with a very broad range of views, to give you a sense of how many perspectives there are on this at the moment.

The first person to raise concerns about how these drugs potentially affect the reward systems with me was Gregg Stanwood. He said that if this way of thinking about how the drugs work is right, then, over time, taking these drugs 'might be experienced as anhedonia'. This is when you have a seriously reduced ability to experience pleasure – or, as he put it, 'blunted reward'. He stresses he doesn't think that is likely, 'but I need to suggest that, theoretically, it's possible'. There have been clear examples of this happening with some pharmaceuticals. For example, if you give people who are experiencing psychosis drugs to treat that condition which work by blocking dopamine (which is a key part of the reward system), then that 'absolutely produces anhedonia, and has negative effects'.

When I asked Patricia Grigson, who had carried out the path-breaking work showing that GLP-1 agonists reduce the use of heroin and fentanyl in rats, about this, she said: 'I think it's a fundamental question.' Your reward system makes you seek out all the things you need in life – like food and sex. 'It's important we tend to our real needs, and with vigour. That's what I think is important to figure out – to make sure people [taking these drugs] are still tending to their real needs with vigour.' But she added that your reward system goes beyond just meeting your basic needs. 'If you think about a triathlete or a marathoner, or any of us who aspire to be the best at whatever we're engaging in – a person who wants to be the best violinist. These things take thousands and thousands of hours of motivation and energy. Are we going to have that? Are we going to interfere with that? If we interfere with that, we'll be in big trouble.' Anhedonia is 'a possible scenario', she said, and she is concerned about it.

But she is reassured that, so far, in both her experiments and in the people taking these new weight-loss drugs, 'it's not interfering, it would appear, with their real needs'. For example, 'in our models, animals are continuing to eat chow, they're just not eating as much of a sweet.'

Max Pemberton shared Patricia's concern. 'If it's just generically dampening all of your reward pathways, are we going to produce a lot of people that feel a bit dysthymic, who are going around with a healthy weight but not really enjoying work, or their kids, or whatever? I literally don't know … This would be my concern. I wonder – [let's say] I'm a new mum, and I want to lose my baby weight. I start taking Ozempic. We have no idea – how does that work when you're imprinting, you're baby-bonding? There's clearly a built-in evolutionary neurological basis to that.' Similarly, when I asked about these risks, Christian Hendershot, who studies the drugs in North Carolina, said: 'That definitely comes up … Some people do report an increase in negative mood, negative affect when they're taking these medications … I think there's a possibility that reward that's derived from natural sources could also be dampened … I think it's something to watch out for.'

In July 2023, the European Medicines Agency – the regulator for all medical products in the European Union – raised another safety signal for Ozempic. They warned it was possible that in some people it increases thoughts of suicide and self-harm. This is now being investigated. Shortly afterwards, the British medical regulator also opened an investigation based on the same warnings.

The proponents of the drug say it doesn't take much to trigger a safety signal – in this case, it was three patients in Iceland who became suicidal after taking it. By September 2023, though, this had grown to more than 150 reports across Europe, while the FDA in the United States had received 96 reports of people developing suicidal thoughts after taking the drug. Most safety signals, as I mentioned before, turn out to be false alarms: there are – sadly – suicidal people in the population, and some of them are going to be taking all sorts of drugs; it doesn't necessarily mean the drug caused the suicidal impulse. But the critics of the drug say that the first murmurs that fen-phen caused heart problems were equally small – a few doctors in Fargo, North Dakota, noticing a handful of patients having problems. This revelation eventually caused the whole house of cards to fall. Could these drugs bring with them a wave of depression?

Some other scientists who have thought seriously about these questions do not believe there is any reason to be concerned. When I asked Heath Schmidt, who has been studying these drugs for years, about this, he said: 'We haven't seen it with any of the measures that we've done in our animal models. I'm also not aware of any reports from diabetics or people taking these drugs for weight-loss management that they're no longer interested in sex … I haven't seen any concrete evidence that it's producing anhedonia.'

I also put this concern to the companies making these drugs. Novo Nordisk said they 'will continue to monitor reports of adverse drug reactions, including suicide and suicidal ideation, through routine pharmacovigilance and in cooperation with local health authorities. In the U.S., [the] FDA requires medications for chronic weight management that work on the central nervous system, including Wegovy and Saxenda, to carry a warning about suicidal behavior and ideation. This event had been reported in clinical trials with other weight management products. Novo Nordisk is continuously performing surveillance of the data from ongoing clinical trials and real-world use of its products and collaborates closely with the authorities to ensure patient safety and adequate information to healthcare professionals. Novo Nordisk remains confident in the benefit risk profile of the products and remains committed to ensuring patient safety. The long-term data from [the clinical trials known as] SELECT published recently with Semaglutide exposure over 39 months is reassuring that there is no increase in the risk of psychiatric disorders with Semaglutide 2.4 in comparison with placebo.'

Eli Lilly declined to comment.

~

I kept coming back to what seemed to me to be the key question about the drugs' function: if they work by repressing my reward systems, how can they tell the difference between something that's bad for me – eating that second box of Chicken McNuggets – and something that's good for me, like going for a run? Elisabet Jerlhag, who did the key experiments giving GLP-1 agonists to alcohol-glugging rats, told me that these drugs seem to be selective. They found in their experiments that the drugs reduce the amount of dopamine triggered by alcohol, but *not* the amount of dopamine released overall. 'If you had a drug that reduced dopamine per se, then you would expect that drug might [produce] anhedonia – that you are unmotivated. You don't feel any pleasure.' But that's not what they saw. The rats still scampered around, had sex and ran in their wheels. 'In our models at least, it doesn't affect activity per se, or dopamine per se.' It looks like it is 'a drug that only blocks what's excessive'.

I was puzzled by this. Let's say I'm Elton John and my primary source of pleasure comes from creating great music. How does a drug working on my reward system know to suppress eating jam sandwiches but not to suppress jamming? 'Yeah. We don't know,' Heath Schmidt said. 'Honestly, I think that's a great question … That's why we're doing a lot of these mechanistic studies in the brain, to try to figure out what exactly is going on.' When I asked Elisabet the same question, she said 'there are no studies' looking at how it might affect love of music. 'So I don't know.' But given how many people take GLP-1 agonists for diabetes and obesity, 'I think it would have been reported if you're a musician and you don't have reward from that any more. I haven't read any reports on it. But I think, of course, you have to be careful.'

It all comes down to how selective the effects of the drug on the brain really are. Elisabet said that the brain certainly has the capacity to be selective in this way. 'When you have a natural, normal concept of rewarding things that you like,' such as eating heathy food, or listening to music, your dopamine system works as it should. But when you become addicted, to overeating or alcohol or cocaine, 'these addictive behaviours hijack the mesolimbic system [in your brain]. Then, it's different. It acts on the system differently.' The brain 'has been established to separate' these different states, so it's possible the drugs can distinguish between them too. But for the scientific community, 'you have to study it much more, because you're in the beginning now of understanding how it works.'

~

As I spoke with more scientists and dug into their research, some of them told me that I shouldn't be worried about this problem, because my concerns come from the fact that I have been thinking about it in the wrong way. They asked: What if these drugs do *not* work by dampening the reward system after all? What if something else is going on in your brain?

I learned that alongside the theory about reward systems, there are at least two other, different ways of thinking about what these drugs do to our brains. I was taught the first theory from Aurelio Galli, who is the director for Gastrointestinal Biology Research at the University of Alabama at Birmingham. He was one of the first scientists to identify GLP-1 receptors in the brain. He told me that of course dialling down the reward system would be bad. 'Can you imagine a life without reward? You would not be able to survive. You would not be able to live, or at least live well. You're not going to take care of your kids if their smile would not reward you and make you happy. Reward is part of everything we do.' But he doesn't believe that is what these drugs are doing. 'I'm not so sure that it is dampening it. I would be careful. I think that it is *resetting* it,' to 'proper or better neurotransmission in the brain.' It's a little like restoring one of your electronic devices to the factory settings. From this perspective, obesity is the unnatural brain state, and these drugs take it back to a healthy state. His hunch is that the drugs 're-establish a normal pathway. That is how I think.'

Dr Clemence Blouet mooted a similar theory. As I had learned earlier, many scientists believe your body has a natural set point at which it tries to maintain your weight – but as you gain weight, your set point rises, and it tries to keep you at that higher weight. She told me that the drugs 'might lower the set point. It's like [they] lower the temperature at which you maintain your health.' After this resetting, your brain and your body stop fighting to keep you at a higher weight, and allow you to go down to a lower weight without tormenting you with all these mechanisms – a slower metabolism, greater hunger, less energy – that are designed to drag you back.

The second theory is that the drugs don't work primarily by suppressing the reward system, but instead by boosting a different system in your brain. Paul Kenny said that to understand what he thinks is happening you need to know 'there are these two parallel systems' in your brain. There's the reward system, which gets you to seek out things that make you feel good. But at the same time, 'you've got a parallel system – the yang to the yin of the reward system – which is the aversion system. They tell you to stop, [that] what you're doing is bad for you, could kill you, or is not life-sustaining.' This is what kicks in when your body tells you to stop eating, or smoking. These two systems 'have to work together. All too often, when we think about disorders of consumption – like obesity or drug addiction – [we focus on] the reward end of things. But there's also an aversion end. When you're using drugs, they also activate brain aversion systems that tell you – "Hey, you should stop doing this." '

This is the system Paul suspects is boosted by these drugs. 'It's turning on the satiety systems,' he said. 'We know much less about the aversion systems than reward systems. If I was to speculate, I'd say what these GLP-1 agonists are doing is not necessarily modifying the reward systems. They're really turning up the aversion systems – the systems that say "stop doing that. You shouldn't be doing that", so you get the satiety response.' If Paul is right, this would make the potential harms of a reduced reward system – like depression – much less likely.

If this is the case, these drugs would not be working primarily on the reward system, but on much broader areas of the brain. What, I wondered, would be the potential risks of that?

One area these drugs affect is the hindbrain. So I asked Clemence Blouet: What are the risks of altering the hindbrain? What else does it do? 'It's important for taste processing. It's involved in the autonomic control of blood pressure, heart rate and gut motility.' Another part of the brain these drugs affect is the arcuate nucleus of the hypothalamus. I asked her about the potential risks of messing with it. She said this part of the brain is important for memory processing, and 'you can always speculate that when you hit the system very hard with a drug long term, you might change the way these pathways are organised, your connections, and the way they sense other signals. Yes, it's possible. I don't think we know enough about this.' She stressed that raising these effects is 'highly speculative'. We really don't know.

Sometimes, the risks of taking a drug that affects the brain only emerge many years after people start to take them. Gregg Stanwood raised this concern with me gingerly. 'I don't want to cause alarm. I hesitate to bring it up with you at all as you're writing this,' he said. 'But I do think there are issues around the biology of these systems that we still need to address.'

With what felt like a deep breath, he said: 'So I have concerns about women of childbearing age who aren't pregnant, who may become pregnant.' Being on one of these medications 'might have deleterious effects on their pregnancy and on babies' development. I'm mostly concerned about the third trimester, based on the receptor activity' in the brain of the foetus.

If the mother is taking these drugs, then they could affect the development of the brain of the baby inside her, at a crucial and formative stage. 'I guess my concern – worst-case scenario – is you alter these developing circuits in the brain that are involved in reward systems. You might create an alteration in developmental trajectory of these kids where, as they grow up, their brains might not respond [normally] to endogenous rewards – whether we're talking about food, drink, sex, gambling, video games. So these individuals might become more, or less, responsive.'

The reason he is worried about this is because of a different set of scientific discoveries. He said I should read the long-term studies that followed the children of women who were exposed to chemicals in the environment (like heavy metals or dangerous plastics), and also the studies of the children of women who used drugs during pregnancy. 'At birth,' he said, 'we don't see much [difference] in offspring from women exposed to some pretty deleterious things. But around school age, we start to see some issues creep in that can be very difficult to treat. Some of those issues involve the reward circuits – increased prevalence of impulsivity and attentional dysfunctions.' It could contribute to a 'rise in substance use'. He stressed: 'So again, I want to be really cautious about it, but the potential is there to do harm.' However, he added, 'it could go in the other direction. Maybe it would be protective. Maybe it would increase resiliency in the system as well. We simply don't have the data to know.'

~

I put this concern to the drug companies that make these medicines. Novo Nordisk said that anyone who was pregnant was excluded from their clinical trials, so there is 'limited' data about how it affects them, but 'these medicines should not be used during pregnancy'. They directed me to part of their official prescribing advice, which says: 'There are limited data with semaglutide use in pregnant women to inform a drug-associated risk for adverse developmental outcomes … Based on animal reproduction studies, there may be potential risks to the fetus from exposure to semaglutide during pregnancy. Ozempic should be used during pregnancy only if the potential benefit justifies the potential risk to the fetus. In pregnant rats administered semaglutide … structural abnormalities and alterations to growth occurred.'

Eli Lilly declined to comment.

~

After learning all this, it was clear to me that we need to think about these drugs very differently from the oversimplified story that has been offered to us up to now.

When you take them, you are not just changing your gut. You are changing your brain. You are changing your mind.

It felt like a deeper and more intimate transformation – and a less predictable one.

8

What Job Was Overeating Doing for You?

The five reasons why we eat – and what happens when they are taken away from us

After everything I had learned about how these drugs affect the brain, I wondered again about my own low mood since I started taking them. Were they dampening the reward centres of my brain? It's possible. Or maybe my low mood was being caused by other things happening in my life at the same time that had nothing to do with Ozempic. But then I learned there was another set of reasons that might explain why I felt this way.

It could be that taking these drugs was not primarily affecting me biologically – but instead, they were affecting me psychologically.

I began to dig into this, and I learned that there's scientific evidence for at least five reasons why we eat. Slowly, I realised that for me, almost all of them were disrupted by Ozempic.

As I began to dig into this, I discovered something sobering. It's only when your eating habits are taken away from you that you understand the job they were doing for you all along.

~

The first reason is the most obvious: we eat to sustain our bodies. We have a physical need for food, and without it, we become weak and irritable, then we become sick. If you had asked me before I started researching this book why I ate, I would have given this as the overwhelming reason. But then Ozempic stripped me down to the core physical function of eating, and it dawned on me how little of my relationship with food had been driven by this urge. Before Ozempic, I ate around 3,200 calories a day. Then, when I ate only to keep my body going, I got by perfectly well on 1,800 calories.

The second reason why we eat is equally obvious. Food gives us pleasure. If I say to you the words 'chocolate cake', or 'spaghetti bolognese', or [insert your own food porn here], you will start to anticipate the flavour bursting in your mouth, the aftertaste, the ecstasy. Most of the people I knew who were taking these new weight-loss drugs told me that their pleasure in food had plummeted, or even vanished. Food felt, to them, joyless and utilitarian – they ate just because they had to, not because they liked it. Many experts are worried about this. Jerold Mande, the Harvard nutritionist, said: 'Pleasure is such an important part of the human experience. Through evolution, what are the two most important things in our existence? Procreation. Reproducing ourselves is based in pleasure. We only need to do that a few times to stay going as a species, and look at how much pleasure is designed around that! But the real human pleasure is eating, because you need to make sure you eat every day. So the body had to create a system of pleasure where you would eat every day and not get tired of it.' In our evolution and deep in our psyches, 'the relationship between food and pleasure is fundamental'. Taking that away is hugely risky, he believes.

He said it's like we've announced '"Let's try this experiment where for half of the population, we're going to remove the primary source of pleasure from their lives, and have them stick with that for the rest of their lives. That's going to really turn out to be a good thing." I don't see how that's possible ... Maybe you'll have a wave of depression that strikes people. Or maybe they'll search for that pleasure in some other way' that's unpredictable and risky. Either way, it 'seems likely to unleash a whole lot of unintended consequences'. Even Jens Juul Holst, one of the scientists who helped develop Ozempic, agrees, telling an interviewer from *Wired* magazine that this loss of pleasure 'may eventually be a problem – that once you've been on this for a year or two, life is so miserably boring that you can't stand it any longer'.

As I read this, I felt sad, but not for the obvious reason. It's not that I had been stripped of the pleasure that comes from food, and I missed it. No: I realised that, to be honest, very little of my eating, even before Ozempic, was driven by pleasure. Sure, I can rhapsodise about the sauce in an In-N-Out Burger, or a good beef pad thai. But I have always eaten too compulsively, too quickly and too busily. The pleasure I took in eating has always been more to create the internal physical sensation of being stuffed, of feeling more than full. Throughout my life, I would almost always rather have eaten quickly from a service station, getting a feeling of being crammed with food, than have eaten slowly in a Michelin-starred restaurant.

I didn't miss the pleasure of eating because it had never been a huge factor in my life. If anything, I think taking these weight-loss drugs slightly increased my enjoyment of food, admittedly from a low base. I only really noticed this when, six months into taking them, I went out for dinner with an old friend who I hadn't seen in a while. She said: 'It's always been a bit strange to eat with you, because you would eat incredibly quickly. You'd shovel so much food into your mouth, so fast, but you never seemed to be enjoying it. Now you're eating much more slowly, and you seem to be actually tasting your food.' As she said it, I realised it was true.

But I suspect I am probably an exception. Many people taking these drugs describe losing their pleasure in eating. Some people find that foods they used to love no longer give them joy. I think it depends where you're starting from: if you are somebody who experiences bliss from food and sees meals as one of the highlights of your day, then these drugs will likely diminish that; but if, like me, you're somebody who stuffs food with little pleasure, then these drugs might actually enhance it.

~

The third reason is that we eat to calm and soothe ourselves. When a group of scientists were investigating comfort eating, one of the people they spoke with said: 'Food is like a sedative to me. It knocks me out, almost like a drug. When I feel any little bit of sadness or anger, I eat. It's almost like being fed as a baby. I will eat and eat until I can't move.' Another person told them: 'Eating stops the process of my brain going. It offers relief from thoughts that might actually be quite uncomfortable.' Nearly 31 per cent of women and 19 per cent of men say they respond to stress by eating in order to feel better.

This coping mechanism has become very widespread. A team of scientists analysed 475 games from the 2004–5 National Football League season. They discovered that if the home team lost, sales of common comfort foods like pizzas surged by 16 per cent the next day. By contrast, if the home team won, consumption of these foods fell by 9 per cent, and among highly committed fans, it fell by 16 per cent. The bigger the pain, the more people hit the food. On the night Donald Trump was elected president in 2016, as the news of each state going into the red column came in, food orders on apps like Grubhub and Uber Eats in blue states massively surged, and people mostly ordered high-fat, high-carb junk. There was a 46 per cent surge in people ordering pizza, a 79 per cent surge in people ordering cupcakes, and a 115 per cent increase in people ordering tacos. Over the next twenty-four hours, as the news sank in, Democrats comfort-ate even more. The day after the election, as the neuroscientist Rachel Herz has pointed out, sales of fried chicken were up 243 per cent in Los Angeles, while sales of mac and cheese were up 302 per cent in Chicago.

This pattern follows after all shocking events. After 9/11, sales of unhealthy snack foods soared too, as they did during the pandemic. It's also true for personal disasters. For men, if you lose your job, your chances of adding 10 per cent or more of your body weight shoot up.

The fact that stress is a big driver of overeating also helps to explain why some groups are more likely to become obese than others. In Western culture, poorer people are often more overweight. That is partly because fresh, healthy food is harder to buy if you don't have money, but in addition it's because being poor is really stressful. I thought about my grandmother, who raised three kids on her own after her husband died young, scrambling through cleaning toilets on her knees all day. She would come home, exhausted, stressed and grief-stricken, and of course she wanted to eat piles of potatoes and chips, rather than a plate of carrots. It also helps to explain why Black people in the US are more likely to be obese: They are living with the stress of living in a racist society, where they are more discriminated against, and in greater danger from the police. This goes for other traumatised groups. During the First World War, it was noticed that lots of women who didn't know the fate of their lovers or husbands gained a lot of weight, and it was even given a term: *Kummerspeck*, or 'fat of sorrow'. Among American soldiers who fought in the Vietnam War and were traumatised by it, 84 per cent are obese – far higher than in the wider population.

In my own life, when I was feeling stressed or sad or angry, I would usually overeat. It wasn't particularly conscious, but it was persistent. A bad day would quite quickly become a high-calorie day. But then Ozempic, almost overnight, took that away. I literally couldn't respond to stress by eating – if I tried, I quickly felt sated, and if I ate beyond that, I felt sick and would throw up. So I just had to sit with the negative emotions. As I reflected on this, I realised I didn't need the more technical-sounding concerns about Ozempic potentially dampening my reward system to explain why I had been feeling so uneasy. One of my primary coping mechanisms had been taken away from me. I couldn't swamp my distress in saturated fats.

In the two years leading up to taking Ozempic, I had gained quite a lot of weight, and it wasn't hard to see why. Between 2020 and 2022, I went through a series of shocking events. I had a suicide in my close family. Separately, a friend of mine was murdered, and I spent a lot of time investigating his murder and the wider serial killings in Las Vegas (the subject of my next book). Oh – and there was a global pandemic that killed millions of people, disrupting the lives of everyone I knew.

All that overeating was doing a lot of work for me. It was acting as a shock absorber. Because I grew up in a crazy and unstable environment, I think I have always taken for granted my ability to soak up stress and keep going. Overeating did a really important job for me. It made it possible for me to go forward when I might easily have buckled. It gave me some padding from externally imposed pain. But it was a solution that, in turn, caused many problems of its own.

On Ozempic, that solution has been stripped away. I was leaner, and healthier. I was also naked before the pain.

~

Deprived of the ability to comfort-eat, something odd happened. Even at my fattest, I had never been a big fan of sugary treats – my weaknesses were always carbs and fried food. But on Ozempic, I developed a sweet tooth for the first time. I bought packs of sweets, which I hadn't done since I was twelve years old. By doing this, I discovered there was a way I could hack the Ozempic and still comfort-eat a little. I bought a pack of marshmallows and ate them all, and found that – presumably because they are so light and fluffy – they didn't trigger the satiety response that Ozempic normally caused to kick in. I was able to get a buzz of sugary comfort without feeling sick.

You'll have to watch yourself with these marshmallows, I thought to myself.

~

Speaking of comfort food, all throughout writing this book, I have repeatedly mistyped 'fried chicken' as 'friend chicken'. I don't think you need to be Freud to decode that slip.

~

The fourth reason we eat is one that has become unfashionable, but I think it is worth exploring. It is because we are re-enacting the psychological patterns we learned as children around food. This is easier to understand when you learn the story of how it was discovered.

In 1934, a German-Jewish psychoanalyst named Hilde Bruch arrived in the United States, relieved to be beyond the reach of the Nazis at last. Quite quickly, she noticed something in her new life that surprised her. Even back then, there were more obese kids in the US than she had ever seen in Germany. She wondered why.

Under Hitler, obesity was explained entirely in 'racial' terms – it was often presented, grotesquely, as a sign of racial inferiority, with diabetes in particular explained as a 'Jewish disease'. In the US, it was seen at the time as entirely the result of malfunctioning genes – a child was overweight purely because there was something wrong with their biology. This wasn't as racialised as under the Nazis, but to Hilde, it seemed equally simplistic. She (rightly) believed genes played some role in obesity, but it seemed unlikely that they explained everything. She wanted to find out what else might be going on.

She began to suspect that, at some level, there was something going on in the psyches of people who overeat, and if it could be understood, she might be able to help them. So she got a job working in the obesity clinic at Columbia Presbyterian Medical

Center in New York, and over three years, she got to know hundreds of families who had overweight kids. One day, a boy named Saul was brought in by his mother. He was fourteen years old, five foot five and weighed three hundred pounds. The standard script that the clinic had been following for years was clear: tell the boy to eat less. Tell the parents he's genetically cursed. The end. Hilde wanted to try something different, so she started to ask questions about the boy's life.

It turned out something had happened to Saul. His parents were Orthodox Jews, and their first two children were girls. Saul's mother really didn't want to have any more kids, but his father desperately wanted a son, and wore down his wife. In the weeks and months that followed Saul's birth, his mother found it hard to connect with the baby at all. She struggled to even feed him. Then, when he was about four months old, she developed a backache – one for which no doctor could find a cause. She said that as a result of her bad back, she couldn't lift the baby, so he was left in his crib, where he would scream and thrash. She discovered there was one way to silence him – to shove cookies into his mouth. Given this rush of sugar, he would be silent for a while – but not for long. She started to shovel more and more cookies into him. Hilde explained: 'Saul's weight was normal at eight months, but he had become decidedly chubby at ten months.'

This sounded to Hilde like a story not of a genetic disorder, but of a depressed and deeply unhappy mother who was unable to cope with a baby she never wanted. She numbed her baby with food and, over time, Saul learned to numb himself in the same way. Hilde started to suspect, as she wrote: 'This early "programming" of his regulatory centers became his permanent pattern.'

Hilde was slowly pioneering the application of psychotherapy to obese children like Saul. She argued that the parents of these kids often required extra help to understand their children's needs and to meet those needs. The earlier you can help them, the better the results. She believed that from the moment babies are born, they are trying to communicate to their caregivers what they want by the only tools they have, screams and cries. When things go well, the parent learns to understand what the baby's needs are, and meets those needs, and the child learns to understand and meet her own needs. But sometimes that goes wrong – and one of the places where that can happen is in relation to the baby's hunger.

Parents feed their children differently. Some learn how to see when their child is hungry, and feed her then, and only then. That child will learn, slowly, over time, to eat primarily to meet her own physical hunger. But some use food much more broadly. They can be like Saul's mother, using food as, in Hilde's words, 'the great pacifier, without regard for the real reason for the child's discomfort'. Under stress themselves, they use food to shut the baby up, or they withhold food as a punishment. When this happens, often the child 'will grow up confused and unable to differentiate between various needs'. The child learns to eat not just when she is hungry, but to deal with all sorts of other feelings, like being anxious, or bored, or angry.

We are sensitive to the way we were taught to think about food when we were very young, Hilde believed, and we are prone to act it out unconsciously throughout our lives. As I read through her work, I couldn't help but think of my own childhood. I had a father who tried to encourage me to eat healthily, but the only tools he used were shame and force, because that is all he had been shown as a child himself. I had a mother and grandmother who would then smuggle me unhealthy food, behind his back. So I learned – at a deep, pre-rational level – to associate healthy food with shame and fear, and unhealthy food with love. It seemed ludicrous and embarrassing, as a 44-year-old man, to realise I was still acting this out, all these years later, long after I had learned to see how dysfunctional that environment was. But I could see that it was true: the unconscious reflexes I developed in this old story meant something was happening when I took these weight-loss drugs. When Ozempic pushed me towards eating in a healthier way, I experienced it not as a joyful liberation, but as a frightening and slightly shameful deprivation. I felt like I was being deprived not just of junk food, but of love. I felt, in fact, like I was being punished.

Psychological explanations for obesity like Hilde's have gone out of fashion, like psychoanalysis itself. It's certainly true that these explanations were overstated for a while – in 1959, after Hilde and others popularised them, the *New York Times* claimed that psychological problems were responsible for 90 per cent of obesity, which is a big overstatement. But we have swung too far the other way. How could something as basic to human beings as eating not be profoundly shaped by, and intertwined with, our psyches? How could understanding those underlying psychological drivers not help us?

In the 1970s, a scientist named Leann Birch at Penn State University was inspired by Hilde, and decided to use modern scientific methods to figure out if the psychoanalyst's hunches had been right. She conducted over thirty studies over the years, aiming to discover whether, using Hilde's core ideas, you could actually reduce childhood obesity. To give an example of one of her studies, her team at Penn State Children's Hospital took a group of 279 first-time mothers, and split them into two groups. The first were given intensive support in learning how to tell the difference between when their kids were crying because they were hungry, or overstimulated, or distressed, or tired. Ian Paul, a doctor who worked on the study, told me that the mothers and babies were taught that 'food should be used for hunger', not for solving these other problems. The mothers were gently guided to feed their kids when they were hungry, and to respond to the other situations not with food, but with different techniques. The second group were not given any of this training. Leann then followed these parents and babies over time, to see if there was any difference.

The children of the mothers in the first group turned out to be *half* as likely to become overweight or obese. This and other studies conducted over the years suggest that Hilde was right: how our parents read our signals of hunger and respond to them shape us deeply, and can play a significant role in our later weights. Based on this growing body of evidence, more and more experts now recommend teaching 'responsive parenting' to all mothers and fathers.

~

The fifth reason we eat is the one that might be the most challenging to take on board – it was for me, anyway. But it is, for many people, very important. It is that being overweight can psychologically protect you.

I first learned about this from Dr Vincent Felitti, a scientist who has made a series of breakthroughs. I got to know him in San Diego in 2016 when I interviewed him for one of my previous books, *Lost Connections*, which is about depression. When I was thinking about Ozempic, I found myself reflecting on his story and listening again to our interviews. I'd like to briefly restate a little of what I wrote in that book, so I can explore how it helped me to think about these new drugs, and why they made me feel so strange at first.

In the early 1980s, Vincent was approached by Kaiser Permanente, the big not-for-profit medical provider in California, with a problem. Obesity was rising dramatically, and it was both harming people's health and swelling Kaiser's costs. None of the solutions they tried were working. They gave people diet plans and exercise programmes, but their weight continued to increase. So they offered Vincent a big pot of money to do blue skies research. They wanted him to figure out what could reverse this dangerous trend. He agreed to do it, and immediately felt stumped. What could he do? What should he try? He started to work with a group of 286 severely obese people, and one day, he had an idea that seems, at first glance, to be quite stupid.

What if severely obese people literally just stopped eating? Provided we gave them vitamin shots so they didn't develop scurvy or malnutrition, would they just burn through the fat supplies in their bodies and lose weight?

With a lot of careful medical supervision, he tried it – and incredibly, at first, it seemed to work. There was a typical patient who he called Susan (to protect her medical confidentiality), who went from being 408 pounds (29 stone) to just 132 pounds (9.4 stone). Her family told him he had saved her life. She seemed thrilled. But then, one day, something unexpected happened. She started to obsessively eat again, and her weight began to balloon back up. Vincent called her in and asked her what had happened. She felt ashamed and looked down. She said she didn't know. He asked her about the day she started to overeat again – did anything happen that day that didn't happen on any other day? It turned out something had happened that day that had never happened to Susan before. A man had hit on her. Not in a nasty way – in a nice way. But she'd felt terrified, and started to obsessively overeat.

That's when Vincent asked her something he had not thought to ask any of his patients before – when had she started to put on weight? It was when she was ten, she said. He asked: Did anything happen when you were ten that didn't happen in any other year? After a long silence, she told him that was when her grandfather started to rape her.

Vincent interviewed everyone in the programme and discovered that 60 per cent of them had made their extreme weight gain in the aftermath of being sexually abused or assaulted. 'I was incredulous,' he told me. It seemed bizarre. Why would sexual abuse lead to weight gain?

Susan gave him the answer. 'Overweight is overlooked,' she said, 'and that's the way I need to be.'

Sitting there, Vincent wondered for the first time: 'What are the benefits of being fat? We all know the risks – you can get a government pamphlet on those.' But what does it do that's positive? One of the benefits, he realised, is that 'it's sexually protective'. You attract less predatory male attention if you are overweight or obese, and Susan had a very good reason to want to live with that extra layer of safety. It is not surprising, then, that when Susan's weight plummeted, she felt incredibly frightened and anxious. She had talked to Vincent about it 'coming off faster than I can handle it'. He told me: 'What we had perceived as the problem – namely, major obesity – was in fact very frequently the solution to problems that the rest of us knew nothing about.'

The writer Roxane Gay writes about this in her moving memoir *Hunger*. When she was in her early teens, she was gang-raped by a group of young boys, led by somebody she believed was her friend. In the aftermath, 'I began eating to change my body. I was wilful in this … I knew I wouldn't be able to endure another such violation, and so I ate because I thought if my body became repulsive, I could keep men away.' Later in her life, if she lost weight, she would 'worry about my body becoming more vulnerable as it grows smaller. I start to imagine all the ways I could be hurt.'

Vincent told me there are other ways obesity can protect people. It can, for example, lower people's expectations of you – because of stigma, they will expect less of an overweight person, which can relieve pressure on you.

I think it carried out a role for me too, although my experiences were not as extreme as Susan or Roxane. I am a ferociously self-critical person – left to my own devices, without constant stimulation and connection and activity, my mind can easily flip into a frenzy of condemning myself. Being overweight perhaps provided me with a safe-ish outlet for my self-criticism. When those negative thoughts came, I could turn them onto my body, and criticise myself for my eating. This wasn't a pleasant process, but it provided a familiar race-track on which my negative thoughts could be allowed to run. Once that racetrack was taken away, and my negative thoughts couldn't be focused on my body, they started to gallop more widely across my life.

~

Losing weight made me physically healthier. But for all these underlying reasons, it also made me more psychologically vulnerable at first.

What, I wondered, will be the effect when millions of people are deprived of the psychological protections they get from overeating? There's one body of scientific evidence that could potentially give us an early clue.

Earlier in this book, I explained that I had learned about the extraordinary physical benefits that come from bariatric surgery, which is the closest thing humans have had to these new weight-loss drugs until now. People who have this surgery experience a massive fall in the risk of heart attack, diabetes, hypertension, inflammation – the list goes on and on. That's why most people are glad they did it, and a majority see an improvement in their mental health too. But for a small but significant minority, they experience two severe psychological side effects – ones which might make the debate about how these weight-loss drugs affect depression and addiction even more complex.

I discussed the first of these effects with Robin Moore, who works in the not-for-profit sector in Toronto. One day, she realised she had reached 303 pounds (21.6 stone), and she felt total despair. She told me that when it came to food, 'I was a slave to it. Literally. If your eyes are open, it's a constant battle of – what can I eat now? What am I going to eat next? How am I going to get it? Am I going to be safe to eat? Are people going to be around,' judging her for eating? The food made it possible for her to feel 'numbed. Totally. I was being numbed and removed from life.'

She had some sense how she had ended up living this way. When she was eleven, growing up in the suburbs of Toronto, she had been raped, and she had never told anyone. She found it very hard to trust men, or let them come close to her. She ate to cope with the aching loneliness. 'The only thing that feels good when you're in a spiral like that is to eat more,' but 'it's a spiral downwards. You gain weight, people treat you really badly, you feel worse, you want to comfort yourself by eating more. Down and down.'

She finally turned to bariatric surgery because, she told me, she felt 'there's nothing else. I was just absolutely powerless and frantic and so full of self-loathing.' In April 2001, she had the operation. As she came round from the surgery, she saw her mother, smiled, and said: 'I'm on my way.' In the next six months, she lost ninety pounds (6.4 stone). 'It was so fast. I would have three bites of something and I'd be full. It was just incredible.' She joined a running club, and started dating men for the first time. 'I've struggled with relationships with men my whole life. You want it, but you're terrified.' Now, she began to have a sex life, and to discover the joy of it. 'The surgery to me was a gift – an absolute gift.'

But then something happened. Robin had never been a heavy drinker, except for a short phase when she was in her teens. When she went out with her friends from the running club, she would order a glass or two of red wine. Very quickly, it began to escalate. In the space of a few months, she realised she was drinking three bottles a day. 'I just went right off a cliff. It was disastrous … I lived centrally in the city and I was working out by the airport, and I used to take the subway and a bus to where I worked. It was a long commute, about three hours a day. I thought to myself – okay, I'm doing all right because I can get to work two days out of five not drinking' on the journey out there. She started secretly drinking at work. One Thursday morning, her colleagues noticed she was slurring. She was sent home in a taxi, and told to see her doctor. 'I was absolutely smashed,' Robin recalled. On the Monday, she was fired.

Roughly one in ten of the people who have bariatric surgery develop an addiction to alcohol, or gambling, or shopping, or drugs, in the aftermath. They are often referred to as 'addiction transfers' – where somebody's obsession with being comforted by food shifts to being comforted by another compulsive behaviour. Carel Le Roux, the doctor who has been involved in both bariatric surgery and the development of Ozempic, told me: 'We see that a lot with bariatric surgery. A lot.'

He believes it is because for those patients, overeating has performed a psychological function, and afterwards, there's 'this hole, this space, left in their reward areas that's not filled any more. We try to encourage people to fill that space, for example, with exercise. I think most people fill that space with shopping. They become addicted to shopping' for new clothes for their new bodies. 'I think that's all very acceptable. But there's also socially unacceptable ways – gambling, or sex addiction, or alcohol addiction in a small number of patients … That's something that is real, and people suffer.' The nutritionist and eating disorders expert Jessica Setnick told me that this happens because surgery 'doesn't solve any emotional problems. It doesn't solve habitual behaviours. It doesn't solve learned behaviours. Absolutely not. If you're a person who copes with stress by eating, and then you can no longer eat, you have to find another way to cope with stress – and there's no guarantee that it's a healthy method … If someone takes away the way that you use to feel better, of course you're going to find some other way to feel better. It's obvious. You're not just going to tolerate feeling bad. That's not the human way. We're going to either look for something else or get really depressed and suicidal.'

There may be a physical component to this. After bariatric surgery, your body metabolises alcohol differently – you get drunker, quicker, and it stays in your system for longer. But there is always a large psychological component to any addiction. After surgery, some people believe that losing weight will solve all their problems and set them free to become who they really are. Carel said that many of them then realise 'I have the same job, and I drive the same car, and I live in the same house, and I have the same partner. Actually, it wasn't the disease of obesity that made my life terrible. It was all this other stuff.' For others, the increased attention from potential sexual partners triggers memories of sexual abuse, as it did for Vincent Felitti's patient Susan.

After she was fired, Robin went to Alcoholics Anonymous, and discovered the power of healing and healthy connections. By the time I got to know her, she had been abstinent from alcohol for seventeen years, and she was glowing with obvious good health, both physically and psychologically. For her, the surgery and the alcoholism led her to confront the underlying issues that had been driving her all along, and to find her way to connection. But this doesn't happen with everyone. For some, it gets even darker.

~

There is another psychological side effect of bariatric surgery. It can often overlap with addiction, but it's different. I discussed it with somebody who had seen it up close. (I have changed the names of the people involved and some minor identifying details.)

Wilma met her husband Michael in their small town in West Texas in the 1980s, when she was seventeen, and he was twenty-one. He caught her eye because he was very athletic, and played on several sports teams. After they got married, he started to work on an oil rig, and began to gain weight. By the time he was in his early forties, he weighed more than 400 pounds (28.5 stone), but he didn't take any shit about his weight from anyone. One of his colleagues nicknamed him 'Slim', and one day, Michael called him 'Good-Looking' in reply. When the man asked him why he was calling him that, he said: 'Well, I figure if you can lie to me, I can lie to you.'

Wilma loved her husband and didn't raise the issue of his weight with him. She was struck that other people didn't extend the same courtesy to her – they seemed to feel entitled to ask her extraordinarily crude questions about her husband's body, sometimes even asking her if they really had sex.

After Michael had bariatric surgery, he lost half his body weight. People didn't recognise him. When he went out for dinner with Wilma, he joked that people would think she had a new boyfriend. But Wilma started to notice something disconcerting. In their thirty years of marriage, she had rarely seen him seriously drunk. Now he was getting drunk most days. His judgement seemed to be off. It started in small ways.

One day, he was barbecuing a chicken for their dinner, and it caught fire and was charred to a cinder, and he didn't even seem to notice. Another time, she saw him urinating in their driveway. She looked at him and thought: 'This is not my husband. This is a stranger.'

His odd behaviour began to escalate. One night, he came home from a bar stinking drunk, and Wilma asked him how he got back. He said he had driven himself home. That was her limit. She told him that she was leaving him, packed her bags, and walked out.

A few days later, their son came home, opened the garage door, and found that Michael had killed himself.

Following bariatric surgery, a significant minority – 17 per cent – experience depression and anxiety so severe that they need inpatient psychiatric treatment. Carel Le Roux said: 'After bariatric surgery, we [see an] increase [in] suicide fourfold.' The overall risk remains very low – but it goes up dramatically. It seems to happen for the same reasons that some people become addicted. Deprived of the underlying reasons why we eat, they find they cannot cope with life. I asked him if this might happen with the new weight-loss drugs. 'I haven't seen any reports to that effect, but I would not be surprised if it happens,' he said. I thought again about the fact that the European regulators had raised a safety signal on Ozempic, different to the one for thyroid cancer, warning that it may cause an increase in suicide. Could the bariatric surgery suicides be a harbinger of weight-loss-drug suicides?

These insights make the debate about these new drugs, and their effect on addiction and depression, even more complicated. I had already learned that if these drugs work by dampening the brain's reward systems – and it's a big 'if' – then they could have positive effects for addiction, and negative effects for depression. But at the same time, they could be stripping some people of the psychological benefits they get from overeating, triggering *more* addiction and depression.

I asked Wilma if she knew why Michael overate, and why losing those comforts led him to end his own life. 'I don't know,' she said. 'I don't know what it was. He never shared.' We were both silent for a moment.

~

My experiences were far less extreme than these bariatric surgery patients. Most of the time on Ozempic, I was pleased with the amazing physical progress, with a recurrent undertow of loss for the ways overeating had soothed me.

But I now believe that everyone taking these drugs should ask themselves at the start: What job is overeating, and being overweight, doing for you? What did you get out of it that's positive and improves your life? You need to think about this with ruthless honesty, because when you take away the overeating, those issues will likely play out for you in some other way.

Of course, there are lots of people whose overeating isn't primarily driven by these psychological issues, but instead mainly by environmental and biological factors; for them, the psychological issues will be minor. But for some others, they will be huge. One day, in the seventh month of taking Ozempic, I felt immensely stressed about a serious problem, so I went to KFC and ordered a bucket of fried chicken, and I could only eat a single chicken drumstick. As Colonel Sanders beamed down at me from the wall – as he had throughout so much of my life – I felt lost.

I went to visit my friend Judy, who had earlier talked me out of quitting these drugs when I worried it was contrary to my values. I told her that now I felt taking Ozempic was triggering too many psychological issues, and that I should stop taking it. She put her hand on mine. 'Johann, it's not triggering these issues. These issues were there all along. It's just bringing them into view.'

She leaned forward. 'I don't believe that Ozempic is the drug that caused this problem. I think it's just reduced your ability to use the drug you were using to soothe yourself for so long – food. You can stop taking the Ozempic, sure. Stop if you want to. But these issues will still be driving you. I think the answer isn't to stop taking these drugs and slide back to where you were. It's to use this as an opportunity to figure out why you ate in the way you did, and change it. You can disentangle all these different reasons why you eat and understand them. For every one of those underlying psychological reasons why you ate, you can find better solutions.'

She said that my job now was to 'change from thinking of food as something you use to change your mood and your emotions, to thinking of it as something that is a form of nutrition and fuel that you put into your body. Try to imagine food not being about what you put in your mouth but what you put into your central nervous system, what you put into your organs, what you put into your muscle tissue, what you put into your skin, what you put into your gut. Think of that as its destination – rather than your mouth and your emotions as the destination.'

She leaned back. 'If you can make that change, you can learn to eat when you're hungry, and to nourish your body, and to actually receive pleasure from your food. I think that's your task now.'

I knew she was right – but I had no idea how to do that.

9

‘I Don’t Think You’re in Your Body’

How Ozempic made me realise I had to change

In one study of the effects of Ozempic on weight, the scientists involved discovered something that caught my eye. They followed people over sixty-eight weeks to see what it did to them. Most of them lost a massive amount of weight – but there was a kicker. By the end of the study, their weight had started to slightly tick up again. They were, it seemed, moving back towards being overweight. At that point, the study stopped. It was only a modest average uptick – the typical patient still weighed 14.9 per cent less at the end than they had at the start. But what would the graph have looked like if they had continued the study?

I thought about this in relation to my friend’s mother, Michele Landsberg. When she was diagnosed with diabetes in 2008, her doctor prescribed Ozempic. She told me: ‘It had this unexpected, unanticipated, marvellous benefit that almost immediately my appetite was decreased by at least 50 per cent. I’ve struggled with my weight all my life – up, down, thin, fat. I’ve never had that satiety feeling. I never felt that full. There was no natural curb on how much I would eat at any one meal.’ But then 'miraculously, I felt quite satisfied after having a quarter or a half of the usual meal. So with no effort whatsoever, I lost forty pounds very easily in six months. I had never been so happy in my life. I threw out all my old fat clothes in this giddy wave of euphoria.'

But as the years passed, 'the weight started creeping back', she said. 'It was so slow and incremental, it was easy to fool myself and say, "Oh well, it's just a few pounds, I'll look after it later." ' Yet 'although I continued on Ozempic, that side effect [of weight loss] vanished into the ether.' Although it continued to work for her diabetes, 'I began to overeat again.' She has now, at the age of eighty-four, gained back about two-thirds of the weight she initially lost. 'It is depressing as hell. Very, very depressing.'

We develop some tolerance to most drugs. That's where your body gets used to it, so that over time, it no longer has the same effect on you. It seemed like one possible explanation is that Michele's body developed tolerance for Ozempic.

How typical is Michele's experience going to be for the rest of us? It's possible that she simply gained weight due to ageing and diabetes – so the drug was having the same effect, but her own physiology was deteriorating.

The experts I spoke with had contrasting views on this question. When I told her I was wondering about tolerance, Shauna Levy, the doctor prescribing these drugs for obesity, said: 'I wonder that too. I suspect some people will' develop tolerance, 'just like they do with any other medicine. We're flooding their body with GLP-1. I don't see how we couldn't.' But, she stressed, 'I don't think it's true for everybody … Time will tell.' Gregg Stanwood, the neuroscientist studying these drugs, said the truth is that on this question 'we know very little'. He suggested we might want to compare it to when similar drugs act on similar parts of the body, because we know that in those cases 'these receptors often down-regulate with chronic activation'. That is, if these areas of your body are overstimulated by a drug, over time, that part of your body will often start to work less hard, which evens out the overall effect. He said he doesn't know if this will happen with a drug like Ozempic, but 'I would be surprised if the proteins' like GLP-1 that occur naturally in your gut 'don't down-regulate with extended use of one of these agonists'. He stressed: 'Now, that doesn't mean [the benefits] would go down to zero' but 'it would be less helpful' over time.

Others disagreed. Robert Kushner, who helped develop Wegovy, said: 'We don't have any data suggesting tolerance develops,' and indeed he argued there's evidence that people don't develop tolerance: diabetics taking the drug do not need to take higher and higher doses to keep their insulin at the same levels. This suggests to him that the drug will continue to work consistently over the long-term for most people.

But Jerold Mande, the Harvard nutritionist, reiterated to me that whenever there is weight loss, 'the body fights back.' It activates all sorts of natural mechanisms to push your weight back to what it was – its previous set point. 'Your body is like, I need to gain it back, and I have lots of simple ways of doing it. I'm kind of tired. I don't really feel like going up that flight of stairs. I'm going to start burning a lot less energy. I'm going to start eating a little more.' He is sceptical that these drugs can, in the long term, override these very deep biological drives. His hunch is 'maybe the body doesn't gain it back by five years. Maybe it gains it back by ten years.'

I asked the companies who make these drugs to comment on this question, but they both declined to do so. However, Novo Nordisk reiterated that these drugs have been used for a long time, and have been subject to lengthy clinical trials.

Carel Le Roux says that, once again, we should look at bariatric surgery for our best comparison. 'Somebody with a gastric bypass who weighed 100kg will go down to about 66kg. They lose about a third of their body weight after one year. At two years, they're about 68kg. At three years, they're about 75kg. Then they start stabilising somewhere between 72 and 75 for twenty years. That's the typical slope that you see. There's no reason in physiology to imagine that we're not going to see the same with the drugs.'

We won't know who's right for a while. But the potential implications of this are serious. I realised it's at least possible – and perhaps probable – that these drugs have simply opened a window of weight loss in my life, one that is time-limited, and slowly closing.

So I asked myself: While that window is open, are you going to use this opportunity to change your habits, gain some self-understanding, and learn some skills to live more healthily? Or are you going to squander this opportunity by eating half a cheeseburger instead of a whole cheeseburger – and in a few years possibly end up right back where you were at the start?

~

The truth is that seven months into taking Ozempic, I was banking the benefits of the weight loss, but making almost no other changes in my life. I was eating much less, but I was, frankly, eating smaller portions of the same old shit. Instead of having a whole chicken roll coated in mayo for breakfast, I had a third of one. Instead of having a Big Mac, fries and nuggets, I just had fries. My diet still consisted overwhelmingly of processed and junk food, just less of it. It was progress – but of a limited kind.

Robert Kushner told me that many of his patients were in the same position. 'Some people come in thinking the medication is working and they don't go any further than that. So I force them to reflect. What are you doing with these new sensations? Are you choosing and consuming less ultra-processed foods? Are you having more fruits and vegetables? What is your pattern of eating? Are you having a more plant-based diet? Equally, are you more physically active? Are you doing resistance training? Are you going for hikes? Are you walking your dog?' When I told him I was still eating badly, he smiled sympathetically, and said: 'We know diet quality impacts health. Forget about the drug. We know there's mounds of data that shows that a nutritionally balanced diet, high in fruits and vegetables and reduced in saturated fat and trans fat and meat products, leads to a heck of a lot of [good] health outcomes … To improve your health, you have to go the extra mile. You have to now look at the quality of your diet and your physical activity.'

Whenever I heard this advice, I both knew it to be true and felt totally at a loss about how to implement it. How would I even begin? I find this embarrassing to say, because I think of myself as a competent person – I can travel all over the world investigating complex concepts and making sense of them for large audiences – but when it comes to the basic skill of feeding my body, I had no clue what to do. I had never cooked anything that wasn't made in a microwave. Literally never. Almost everything I ate, unless it was cooked by somebody else, was a takeaway or eaten in a restaurant. When it came to food, I felt like I was the equivalent of an illiterate person who is brusquely handed a copy of *War and Peace* and ordered to read.

I only began to feel less foolish about this after I read the food writer Bee Wilson's wonderful book *First Bite*. In it, she explains: 'Eating is not something we are born instinctively knowing how to do, like breathing. It is something we learn.' We are taught how to eat from the moment we are born – and we can easily be taught to eat the wrong things for the wrong reasons. She adds: 'The reason many find it hard to eat healthily is that we have never learned any differently.' I realised that this was true for me. I had never learned how to feed my body. Right from the start, my eating had been jumbled up with managing my emotions and silencing bad feelings by pumping myself full of processed crap.

But, Bee writes: 'If our food habits are learned, they can also be relearned.'

As I read this, I remembered something my friend Rangan Chatterjee, a doctor, advised me several years earlier: 'Give yourself one month of your life where you try only eating freshly cooked wholefoods. Just one month, where you don't eat anything else. You'll be amazed by how different you feel.'

I realised that to have any chance of following Rangan's advice, I would have to do something humiliatingly basic first: at the age of forty-four, I would have to learn how to cook.

I had no idea where to start, so I asked one of my most competent friends, Rosie, to teach me. I told her I wanted her to imagine she was teaching cooking to a person who had been locked in a cupboard and fed nothing but Burger King all their lives, and hadn't heard of the concept that food could be cooked until today. One evening, I turned up at her house, and on the table, there was a bag of vegetables, and some chicken. 'Today we're going to learn to make two healthy things,' she said. 'The first is a lentil soup, because it's high in protein, low in fat, cheap and really easy.'

She got me to measure out 200 grams of lentils. Then she showed me how to chop an onion, and to slice three carrots and a leek. (Until this moment I believed leeks were a Welsh myth, like goblins or dragons. I was amazed to discover they are real.) 'So this is basically all the ingredients you need, plus vegetable stock and hot water,' she said. She took out a big pan, and asked me to pour some olive oil into it. 'Now wait for it to heat up a little bit.' She demonstrated how to squeeze some garlic into the pan, and I dropped some onions in, hearing a strangely satisfying sizzle. I put in the carrots and the leek, and then the lentils, and kept stirring. She took out some vegetable stock, and then she poured in boiling water. 'Now that will take thirty-five minutes, so while it's cooking, I'm going to show you how to make a chicken stir-fry.' She talked me through how to cook chicken – I was fascinated to discover it could come in non-nugget form – and how to fry it up with vegetables.

We sat down and ate together. It was delicious, but I had no confidence I could follow her instructions on my own. But patiently, as the weeks passed, she kept guiding me, and she taught me how to make other staples, like spaghetti bolognese, and porridge for breakfast.

I wish I could tell you that these lessons came as a revelation, and from then on, I cast aside processed food, and ate nothing but fresh food I prepared myself. But I didn't. I felt embarrassed that I was not good at cooking. But I sensed something deeper was going on – some strange form of resistance to eating well. I kept sliding back to the smaller portions of the old crap I have always eaten.

~

I only began to understand the first glimmers of the reason why when I explained this problem to one of the wisest people I know, the playwright V (formerly known as Eve Ensler), who is best known for writing *The Vagina Monologues* and for leading some of the most important feminist activism of the past forty years. She told me that, as a close friend, she had been worried for a long time that I had an underlying problem, and my poor diet was only a symptom of it. She said I was deeply disconnected from my own body. 'I don't think you're *in* your body,' she said. For years, 'you didn't really think about what you're putting into it, because you're separate from it.' All this stemmed from an underlying error I had fallen into: 'You are treating your body as a thing – a thing that's separate from you … Your whole relationship to your body is: "Get it to work. Get me to do the work I need to do. Serve me, serve me, get me forward." It's a machine that you're pressing on. It's a machine that you're kind of exploiting, to be honest – as opposed to this precious life container we've been given that you have to really honour and nurture and treat well.'

V said she could recognise this in me because she, too, lived in that state for so much of her life. From the age of five, she was sexually abused by her father, and trauma like that, she explained, 'takes you out of your body. Because, for example, in my case, where I was sexually abused and beaten, my body became the landscape of horror. It became the landscape of betrayal. It became the landscape of dread. It became the landscape of everything I wanted to avoid. So I left my body, and it took me years to get back to my body, because trauma occupies you, and then it gets your body – so *you* don't get to be in your body.' She smoked, she drank heavily, she let men treat her badly. In that state, often, 'your body's a burden. You're always at war with your body.' You see it as a 'problem that needs reprimanding and scolding and criticising', and 'it will never be right. No matter what you do, it will always fail… That separation and disembodiment allows for enormous harm to the body, where you can do all kinds of things. You can put on weight that can kill you. You can eat foods that will be toxic. You can not have sleep, which will ruin your whole system. And it's really not even knowing that you're doing that – because you're so detached.'

Her journey back to her body came in an unexpected way. In her fifties, V was so cut off that she didn't even notice that 'I had a tumour the size of an avocado growing in me' until it reached stage four. She was told her chances of surviving were slim. But as she healed after surgery, she began to be in awe of what her body could do. 'What about the fact that I lost seven organs, and my body managed to rearrange itself to accommodate so I could be alive?' She realised: 'My body is a genius. I worship my body.'

With this new-found love, she began to reinhabit her body in the most primal way she could find – by dancing. 'When you are dancing, you move into your body. You feel your body. You move your body to rhythm sounds, and you discover the light and the flow of energy that is in your body, and you become part of that energy flow. So you stop treating your body like a thing that you have to control, and it becomes a part of you that you have to have mercy for – and love. When you get into your body, then you begin to feel compassion for your body,' and you can – at last – begin to hear and feel what it is telling you.

If you want to start treating your body well, she said, you need to learn how to love and value your body. I knew, as soon as she said this, that it contained an important truth – but I didn't know how to translate it into action. I felt like I had been told I needed to learn a language to which I could find no guides. To try to find a way forward, I decided to talk with a scientist who has spent a lot of time studying how people think about their own bodies, and how we can make them healthier.

~

Viren Swami is a professor of social psychology at Anglia Ruskin University in East Anglia in England. He is a lean, bearded man with a cool, watchful gaze. He said right at the start of our conversation that we tend to think about body image as something that only exists when it goes wrong – when somebody becomes anorexic, for example. But, he says, 'everyone has a body image. Everyone has feelings about their body. Everyone has thoughts about their body. Everyone views their body in a particular way.' All of us 'have an inside view of ourselves. If you can imagine a small person sitting inside your brain thinking about your body, feeling your body, and working out what it means to inhabit that body – that's essentially your body image.'

Something disturbing has happened to body image in the past seventy years, he told me. Research in the 1950s found that very few people were unhappy with their bodies. But now 'in the UK, in the US, upwards of 90 per cent of women feel some aspect of negative body image. About 70 per cent of men experience some form of negative body image.' En masse, most of us began to feel our bodies were not good enough. Today, 'the majority of people are discontent with themselves. There is no other field of psychology where we accept that as the norm. If you said 90 per cent of people were depressed, we would have strategies in place to work out why and how we fix that. With body image, we've got to a place I think where we have just accepted this as normal.' We need, he believes, to see this as a crisis, and try to put it right.

There are many reasons why it has happened, but one is simple. A very sophisticated industry discovered it could make a lot of money by making us feel bad about ourselves. To give one example out of thousands, Viren mentioned that the deodorant 'Lynx had this weird advert in the 1990s where a man drops onto a beach. He's really skinny and none of the women like him. Then he puts on his deodorant, and suddenly all the women are flocking to him. That narrative tells you everything about what the advertising industry does. It tells you you are deficient. It tells you you are incomplete.' The man who isn't jacked is an unattractive joke. We are all exposed to hundreds of messages like this every week, so many that we don't even register them. He added bluntly: 'How does this fashion and beauty complex operate? It operates by telling people you are not good enough as you are, and you can rectify those deficiencies by buying some products from us.' As a result, 'everyone is worried about their appearance'.

Then, on social media, we reinforce these ideas on ourselves and the people around us. One of the groups with the most severely negative body images, Viren said, are people who look at social media and think it is showing them what they should look like. 'If I go online and see Daniel Craig and I think "That's what men should look like", and I don't look like that, it's easy to feel bad about myself.' After years of this exposure and reinforcement, we have been left with profoundly distorted abilities to even see our own bodies. One group of scientists gathered a hundred people at St George's Hospital Medical School in London, showed them a box-file, and asked them to estimate its width. They all got it right. Then they asked them to estimate the widths of their own bodies. They were way off, overstating the size of their waists by 25 per cent and their hips by 16 per cent.

Viren has spent years exploring how people can reverse this process and begin to develop positive body images – to appreciate and love their bodies. He said there are several ways to do it. The first step comes from asking yourself a crucial question. What can your body do that you appreciate and value? Most people can right away list some positive things their body does for them. Maybe you like that your body can go for a long walk. Maybe you like that it can lift weights. Maybe you like that it could carry your babies and birth them. Realising and reflecting on this prompts you to 'shift your focus away from what your body looks like, to what your body's able to do.' That is a profoundly healing change. The technical term for what this question stirs in us is 'functionality appreciation': you see your body not as an object that is being constantly evaluated by others, but as yours, giving you gifts.

Another way to improve your body image is by being in nature. Viren conducted five studies that found that when people get out into the natural world, their body image improves significantly. He has a few theories about why this is. 'When you're in nature, you're away from sources that tell you you're not good-looking enough. It also gives you time to feel more self-compassionate.' In nature, most people feel less egotistical, and start to see themselves as part of a wider web of life.

A different and equally powerful way to improve body image is by engaging in what he calls 'embodying activities'. This is anything that makes you feel more situated in your own body: it could be playing football, or dancing, or yoga, or CrossFit. When you start, you often feel – as he put it – 'I'm proud of what my body's able to do'. Crucially, these activities 'promote a greater care for your body'. (There are some exceptions, he added. Ballet dancers, for example, tend to have a worse body image, because there is so much pressure to be a very particular body shape in that world.)

As he said this, I realised how right V had been about my disconnection from my body. Faced with Viren's question – what can your body do that you appreciate? – I was totally stumped for several minutes. I literally couldn't think of anything. Almost everything I valued was in my head – in words, in concepts. After a long think I finally came to the most obvious answer, sex. But beyond that, I really struggled to think of anything else.

Reluctantly, feeling foolish at first, I followed V's and Viren's advice. Over the next few months, I put on cheesy music, and asked people I love – my friends, my relatives, a man I was having a romance with – to dance with me. I felt almost absurdly clumsy and inept. But gradually, moving my body in line with them, I felt a kind of relief and release. We laughed. I felt something growing – a sense of pleasure that my body could do this strange, ridiculous, beautiful thing. As I did, I found that the psychological block I had on cooking fresh, healthy food would lift a little more. I don't want to overstate it – for every day I cooked for myself, I had two days where I slid back to processed food. I have still not been able to follow Rangan's advice about giving myself a whole month with nothing but fresh food. But I feel that, slowly, I am making progress.

~

As I sat at my table and ate a chicken stir-fry I had cooked for myself, I thought: Maybe the effects of Ozempic won't last. Maybe I will develop tolerance, and this suppression of my appetite will cease. If that's the case, then maybe there's still an argument for these drugs. They can open a window in which you can radically interrupt your habits and make a big change. I don't know if we'll be able to use these drugs for ever, but if I can only use them for a short time, I can at least use them to change myself to prepare myself for a future without them.

The next day, I ordered a Double Whopper from Uber Eats. I only ate a third of it. I stared at the rest, slowly congealing in its cardboard box, and thought: This isn't going to be a simple story of linear progress.

10

Self-Acceptance v. Self-Starvation?
What will these drugs mean for eating disorders?

Eight months after I started taking Ozempic, I was FaceTiming with my niece, Erin. In my rational mind, I knew she was eighteen and about to head off to university for the first time – but she's the youngest member of my family, the baby, and to me, she'll always be seven years old. Nobody in the world activates my protective instincts more. She was talking to me from a pub, and she said: 'You've lost so much weight I can actually see your jawline!' She giggled. As I was about to preen at the compliment, her face hardened into a frown. She looked down at herself and said: 'I need to get some Ozempic. Will you buy me some?'

It took me a moment to register that she wasn't joking.

My niece is a normal, healthy weight, and she suddenly looked sad, and contemptuous of her body.

Of all the moments in writing this book, this was the one that most made me feel like I was doing something really wrong. I wondered if by losing weight in the way that I had – and by being so happy about the physical loss – I had contradicted all the messages I had been trying to tell her since she was a toddler. I wanted her to accept herself; to value herself; to not buy into the messages telling women in particular that their bodies need to be shrivelled to have value.

I realised that in the year or so leading up to this conversation, my niece had witnessed a wider change. Unlike when I was her age, there had been some female celebrities in the public eye who weren't skinny – comedians, actresses, reality-show stars. They often talked proudly about being happy with their bodies. But now, suddenly, they had all dramatically shrunk. Very few of them admitted they were taking the new weight-loss drugs, but the only other possible explanation was that there had been an outbreak of dysentery in Malibu. What was this communicating to her? What was I communicating to her?

Thanks in part to these drugs, the glacially slow progress towards presenting a broader range of bodies as acceptable has been slammed into reverse. Some of the most famous women in the world are visibly getting smaller. What will be the effect? There is strong evidence that if you change the kind of women who are represented as beautiful, you change how girls in particular feel about their bodies. For example, in 1966, a survey of high school girls found that 50 per cent of them believed they were too fat. Three years later, in 1969, 80 per cent thought they were too fat. (In reality, only 15 per cent of them were even slightly overweight in medical terms.) What changed? In 1966, a seventeen-year-old model named Lesley Hornby was suddenly and sensationally declared to be the new paragon of female beauty. She was announced as 'the face of 1966' by the fashion press, and became better known as Twiggy. She weighed six and a half stone. After her rise to fame, fashion models shrank – and women's hatred of their own bodies increased.

Would these new weight-loss drugs have a similar effect on girls like my niece? I told Erin that there was no way in the world that I would buy Ozempic for her. She shrugged. She's a resilient person, and it turned out to be a transient desire on her part.

But I wondered how many other girls of a healthy weight were asking the question she'd asked me – and what would happen to them. Exploring this question led me to uncover the twelfth risk that is associated with these drugs.

~

The person I most wanted to discuss this with was Elise Loehnen, a woman who has gone through an incredible transformation in the time I have known her. I first met her in 2017 in a minimalist diner in Los Angeles, when she was the chief content officer for Goop, Gwyneth Paltrow's lifestyle brand. Goop has built a commercial temple of 'wellness', selling people very expensive products and experiences that promise to cleanse and rejuvenate them. Elise was obviously very intelligent, but at first I assumed she was an uncritical part of this world and its ideas. Then something curious happened.

In 2020, Elise was seeing people with Covid on the news, and she thought: 'People are actually dying, and I'm inventing reasons to be unhappy with my perfectly healthy body.' It seemed a form of madness. She left Goop and became increasingly outspoken about the whole philosophy of trying to expensively 'fix' your body – warning that, in her view, this leads women not to liberation, but to self-punishment. She doesn't criticise her former employer, but she is one of the most thoughtful critics of the whole way of thinking that is so dominant in Hollywood, and seeps out from there into much of the culture.

Elise told me there's no point going out for dinner with many of her friends any more, because they're on high doses of Ozempic so they have 'no appetite' and 'no interest in food'. These are women who were already slim when they started, and now they are using the drug to 'completely sever their appetite'. She sits there looking at people pick at their food and thinks: 'Why are we even at dinner?' It looks like, to her friends, 'thinness is so much more satisfying than food'. She shook her head. 'That, to me, is not a price I am willing to pay.'

If you want to know the effect this will have, she believes, you only need to look back to the 1990s, when she and I were teenagers. She went to boarding school when she was fifteen, and around that time, there was an abrupt shift in the kind of body that the fashion industry celebrated. In the 1980s, the star supermodels – Christy Turlington, Cindy Crawford – 'had amazing bodies, but they had, like, bodies', Elise said. 'I'm not saying these women weren't thin, but they didn't look *skinny* … They were tall. They were women. They were not diminutive little creatures.' Then it all changed. Kate Moss was chosen by the fashion industry as the new look. She had a tiny body and appeared almost prepubescent. Breasts were out; emaciation was in. Soon, every model started to look like a starved child. In the sitcom *Absolutely Fabulous*, a fashion magazine editor says: 'If the models get any younger, they'll be chucking foetuses down the catwalk.' In the wake of this, Elise and her friends became obsessed with what she calls 'an unnatural skinniness'. They would look at Kate Moss and think 'we were outgrowing her, outpacing her in our size'. So they started to ask: 'How do you stop yourself from becoming a woman?'

She watched as all her closest friends started to 'winnow away'. They became hyper-regulated around food, severely restricting what they ate and compulsively exercising. 'One was a runner, one was a dancer, one was a rower. I just watched their bodies change.' In that environment, Elise became highly conscious about her own body. 'When I got to boarding school, I was a huge eater, and very active. I would, for breakfast, have two bagels with butter and cinnamon sugar on them.' Although she was not overweight, hearing the other girls constantly critique their own thinner bodies for being fat made her think: 'Whoa, you think *you're* fat?' She started to cut back on eating dramatically.

When an unhealthy image of thinness is promoted to young women, some of them begin to starve themselves – and that creates pressure on other girls to cut back, and on and on the downward spiral goes. 'It was so contagious,' Elise said, 'it's like a quicksand.' But in the age of Ozempic, 'when I look at Kate Moss now, I think – oh, she looks pretty healthy compared to the models that we see today … Our beauty standards have only become more extreme.' She believes that today 'dieting is out, while "elimination" is in'.

She told me you can't think about this clearly unless you reflect on the ways in which women are treated differently from men. Men are allowed a broader range of acceptable body types, from 'dad bods' to 'bears'. When men receive pressure to change their bodies, they usually want to become more muscular – which brings its own challenges and can be taken to extremes, but isn't inherently unhealthy like starving yourself is. Women are given much less permission to find their own place in the world – they have been pressured for thousands of years to make themselves small and to suppress their desires. With Ozempic, they are saying: 'I have no hunger. I have no desire. I will keep myself small at any cost. It is the most important thing to me – more than sustaining myself, or keeping myself alive.' It's a form of erasing yourself. 'Killing our appetites,' she warned in an article, 'seems like a type of death.'

After a lifetime of rejecting and tormenting her own body, Elise said she'd had enough. She didn't want a drug that would tame her flesh. She didn't want to lose her appetite. She decided to live in peace with her body and its longings.

~

We know what happens when these two things collide – the promotion of unnatural thinness, and the existence of a diet drug that makes it possible to restrict what you eat – because it has happened before.

In the 1990s, Ron Wyden, a congressman from Oregon, held congressional hearings on diet pills for the first time. At the time, the most popular kind was a drug that was chemically very similar to the older amphetamines, and acted both as a stimulant and an appetite suppressant. You could get it without a prescription, and as soon as they became available, there was a huge scramble to take it from one section of the population in particular. Vivian Meehan, a nurse who ran the National Association of Anorexia Nervosa and Associated Disorders, told the subcommittee that teenage girls with eating disorders were using these pills on a massive scale. They wanted to starve themselves, and they found they could do it more efficiently using these drugs. The pills, she said, had become 'the means to a devastating eating disorder'.

To explain the effect of these drugs, a twenty-year-old woman named Jessica McDonald took the stand. When she was twelve years old, she said, 'I was very serious about ballet. While I was not in anyway overweight, dancers have a certain look, a certain body type, that I knew I needed to obtain.' The girls at her ballet school obsessively discussed weight and 'everybody was doing something, trying some diet or taking some pill, in an effort to lose weight. It was at this time that I started using diet pills and other products regularly, such as laxatives and diuretics … I wanted to lose weight and I wanted to lose weight fast. I figured that if I could lose weight with one pill, I could lose a lot of weight by taking more pills.' So she would 'take the whole bottle – eighteen to twenty at a time … Needless to say, they didn't make me feel very good. I would get weak, dizzy, nauseous, and, on more than one occasion, I even passed out – sometimes for a minute or longer. I knew something was wrong, but in spite of everything, I continued to take the pills and to lose weight.' She was sure that 'my use of easy-to-obtain, over-the-counter diet products made my problem worse'. They gave her a tool to starve herself that could take her far closer to destroying herself than her willpower alone could ever have achieved. She pleaded with the subcommittee to 'help get diet pills off the shelves. I don't think these pills should be available at all.'

A middle-aged man named Tony Smith, from a town named State Center in Iowa, also took the stand. He said that when his daughter Noelle was ten years old, she started to persistently ask her parents: 'Do you think I'm too fat?' He continued: 'When we went shopping, we would almost always find her at the magazine section, looking at the fashion models or glancing through stories of how to lose weight from various body parts or from some new diet.' She 'came to believe that her success depended on her body image and appearance'. Noelle became obsessed with diet drugs. 'She was constantly sneaking diet products into the house. There was nothing we could do to shut off the supply. Every time we found and took from Noelle a box of diet pills, laxatives or diuretics, she would go to the corner store and buy a new supply. No one ever tried to stop her. No one ever asked why a sixteen-year-old girl was constantly buying diet pills, laxatives and diuretics. I suppose they didn't want to lose the sale.'

On 12 July 1989, Tony and his wife got a phone call from the hospital. Noelle had died of a heart attack. She was twenty years old.

Her dad read out a poem she composed shortly before her death. She had written: 'As I sit / I look down – panicked at the thickness / I've seemed to acquire. / I began to wonder if I'm hungry. / "Oh not yet," I say.'

As I read through this testimony, I kept thinking one thing. The new weight-loss drugs are vastly more effective than anything that Jessica or Noelle could get their hands on. So what will happen when people with eating disorders get hold of them? One of the people who has been most vocal in warning about this is Kimberly Dennis. She is a psychiatrist and the chief medical officer of SunCloud Health, a group that runs eating disorder clinics in Chicago. She believes these new weight-loss drugs are like 'rocket fuel' for people with restrictive eating disorders. Every day in her clinic, she sees people who are trying to starve themselves – and now these new drugs give them the most effective tool for self-starvation that has ever been discovered.

Ozempic arrived at a time when there was already a rising eating disorders crisis. 'During the pandemic,' Kimberly said, 'rates of adolescents admitting to ERs and inpatient units for eating disorder treatment tripled. Skyrocketed.' Now, she thinks, it is going to soar further. This is not, of course, the intention of the companies manufacturing these drugs, who instruct doctors not to give them to people with a BMI below 27. But the sieve through which these drugs are being prescribed is very leaky. To get them, you can see a doctor online, and many of those medics are not checking your BMI effectively via Zoom.

Kimberly also believes these drugs will make it harder for her patients, and people like them, to recover. 'When we try to treat people with eating disorders, one of the things we try to help them to do is get back in touch with themselves, their bodies, their natural hunger cues.' But for 'people who are on these medications, their natural hunger cues are really shut down. So they don't really have that internal "Mmmm, I'm hungry now" feeling. So that's problematic when it comes to treatment.'

There have to be serious warnings about the risks to people with eating disorders attached to these drugs, she said. 'Most general practitioners who are prescribing these medications for weight loss have little or no expertise when it comes to identification of eating disorders.' She thinks these drugs should be prescribed in-person, and by doctors who are knowledgeable about eating disorders and know how to actively screen for them. She fears that people with eating disorders will misuse these drugs to supercharge their starvation.

~

I put this concern to the companies who make these drugs. Novo Nordisk replied that they do 'not promote, suggest, or encourage off-label use, or misuse, of any of our medications. We do our best to ensure patients and doctors are educated about the appropriate use of our products and encourage healthcare providers to only prescribe the right product for the right patient.'

Eli Lilly declined to comment.

~

Another weird thing happened to me after I started taking Ozempic. I talked over everything I was experiencing in my body and learning in my research with my friends. Some of them were thrilled to see me lose weight and start to feel healthier. Most of them were intrigued. A few demanded to know where I was getting it. But one of my closest and oldest friends, who I'll call Lara, reacted very differently.

She seemed snappy and irritable whenever I brought up the topic. If I made the case for the drugs, she would list the arguments against, and if I responded with information I'd been learning, she became hostile and pissy. She had never been overweight, so I knew it wasn't personal defensiveness. It was so out of character that I didn't know how to respond. Then one evening, when she was visiting London, we had dinner together. When I brought up what I had been reading about eating disorders that day, she became angry – significantly more than she had been before – and finally, I asked her what was really going on.

'You're not being honest with yourself,' she said. 'And if you write it like this, then you won't be honest with your readers either.'

I was dumbfounded. She continued: 'You're telling me that everyone using this drug is taking a risk. That they could trigger an eating disorder epidemic in all these young girls. As if we don't already have enough starving young girls. On top of that, you could be giving *yourself* thyroid cancer. You could be giving yourself *all sorts* of problems we don't even know about yet. You go down this long list of the risks. But whenever you acknowledge this danger you're putting yourself and all these vulnerable girls in, you immediately pivot, and talk to me about health. You say you're doing this for your health. You say your motives are to protect your heart. You list the statistics. You say you're weighing it all very carefully. I'm sorry, but I've got to tell you, I think you're kidding yourself. You're not being honest about your motives.'

Lara was speaking with the rush that people have when they are letting out something that's been on their chest for months. 'How much is this really about improving your health? I don't think, for you, it is. Not really. Not primarily. I want you to stop, and really think about it.'

She pushed her plate aside and said: 'I've known you for twenty-five years, and you've never been happy about how you look. You look good. I've always thought you looked good. But you don't think you do. So you're taking this drug – and all these huge risks – to conform to a particular look, an approved look, the most socially approved look. That's why you're doing it. You want to be thin. Those people at that Hollywood party you went to, where you learned about this drug for the first time, and you texted me all excited – they weren't doing this to boost their health. They were already healthy. They had private chefs to cook them the healthiest possible food. They see a personal trainer every day. They were doing it to be unnaturally thin. You aren't taking these risks to have a healthy heart. You're taking them to have cheekbones. That's what you're encouraging this eating disorders epidemic in all these young girls for. That's what you're risking thyroid cancer for. For vanity.'

I let this sink in for a moment. Then, startled, I argued back. I told her that I really was worried about what would happen to my health if I continued at my previous weight. She leaned forward and asked: 'If this drug gave you all the same benefits to your health, but it also gave you boils on your face, would you take it?'

I stopped. I tried to genuinely think about the answer to her question. Would I take it, if it boosted my health, but harmed my looks? She was forcing me to disentangle the motives that had been conveniently tied together all along. I told her honestly: No, I wouldn't. She said: 'Doesn't that tell you something about your motives? If it was really about health, you'd be willing to take a hit to your looks. I think you've used the health argument to rationalise taking a wild risk with your health, and with the young women of this society, so you can look better. If you want to do that, do it. But please – be honest about your motives. Level with yourself.'

I didn't know what to say. Lara is one of the people who knows me best, and I wondered if she was right, and in fact articulating something I had been hiding from myself. Or was she misreading me? 'If you were worried primarily about health, you would be talking to me about exercise, and writing a book about that,' she said. 'Exercise doesn't lead to much weight loss, but my God, it leads to increased health, across the board. But you've barely mentioned exercise. Because it won't make you more conventionally hot. So you talk about drugs not exercise.'

I brought up again the evidence that obesity really does harm your health. She had clearly been thinking about this, and had read up on it to back up what she said next. 'Every time we've talked about this, you do this performance of carefully weighing the risks. You're doing it now, and I can see you've persuaded yourself what you're doing is real. But you've been rigging the calculations all along. Of course being seriously obese is really bad for you. Hannah was clearly really unhealthy' – she had been friends with her too – 'but to talk about you as being in the same category as her is ridiculous. You were a bit overweight. You've always been able to buy clothes in normal shops. You had a BMI of 30. If you look at the evidence about what happens at that weight, it's not good. It makes you more likely to get some health problems. But the big risks kick in at a much higher BMI – 35 or over. That's where people start to get seriously sick. You keep acting like there's two states: there's people with a BMI of 25 or below, and they're fine and healthy, and then you hit 26 and above, and everyone is all in some terrible danger zone together. It's not like that. It's a slope, and you were at the lowest end of the slope. So when you tell me you are weighing the risks of taking these drugs against obesity, I call BS, because you keep taking the dangers faced by severely obese people and acting like they apply to much slimmer people like you, who face totally different odds.'

I told her again about my grandfather's heart attack when he was my age. 'But *you* don't have heart problems,' she replied. 'Look, I'm not saying that it's not sensible for you to take steps to protect your health. Exercise. Eat better. I'll talk to you all day about the psychological problems that led you to overeat. I have a lot of compassion for that. But the idea that, because you were a bit overweight, and because your grandfather died of a heart attack in the 1960s when the ability to detect heart conditions early was totally different, means that now, in 2023, you should be injecting yourself with a risky drug – it's crazy.'

She continued: 'You tell me you're worried about all these young girls who are going to use this drug to starve themselves. But everyone taking these drugs who isn't seriously obese or diabetic is helping to change the culture and make it different – to make it value thinness even more. Girls like your niece get the message loud and clear from that. What they hear is: it's better to be thin than to eat. What was it Kate Moss said? Nothing tastes as good as skinny feels. Maybe it would be worth taking that risk if you really were going to massively boost your health. But you were healthy! No doctor told you you were sick. You didn't have any heart problems, or pre-diabetes. You didn't need a boost to your health.'

I didn't know what to make of any of this. My concerns about my health were real, and Lara was going too far in dismissing them. But she was also forcing me to confront something that was also real. I think, up to that moment, I had overstated how much I was driven by health, and how little by a concern about appearance. I was suddenly acutely aware of how ashamed I had been to be overweight, and how much it felt like a visible sign of failure. Had this skewed my judgement? Was I doing something harmful – to myself, and to other people?

Her tone changed. I could see that her anger had passed. Now she just looked melancholic. 'You know, I thought, at last, in the past few years, we were starting to let people like their bodies, whatever they looked like. It made me feel happy to see it. I hoped you would start to like yours. And now I'm seeing you waging war on your own body. It makes me sad.'

I realised I needed to spend more time researching the movement that has been trying to make us more accepting of our own bodies, whatever they look like. I wanted to know if the answer to Lara's challenge to think more deeply about these questions might lie with them.

11

The Forbidden Body?
What do these new drugs mean for stigma?

In the 1980s, when I was a child, it was taken for granted on television that fat people were shameful – that they were lazy, and greedy, and the deserving butt of jokes. I took this as a given, because I had never heard any different. Then, one day, on a morning TV show, when I was about ten years old, I heard somebody say something new.

Shelley Bovey was one of the first people with any prominence in Britain to talk about fatness in a different way. She has a gentle, lilting voice, and with a tone of quiet dignity, she argued that we needed to stop abusing fat people, and start understanding and respecting them. Her arguments won few supporters at the time, but as the years passed, a movement of people inspired in part by her ideas began to rise up. In the period running up to the launch of these new weight-loss drugs, they started to win significant victories. This movement is increasingly challenging the legitimacy of these drugs, arguing that they are both unnecessary and unjust.

Shelley is seventy-six years old now, and I tracked her down to her home in a village in the south of England. On a summer's morning, she waved to me across a car park outside the train station. Her husband, Alistair, stood protectively next to her. He drove us to her local pub, and we sat there all day, talking over the movement she helped bring to Britain.

~

When Shelley was twelve years old, her teacher told her one day to stay behind after class. As she stood there, wondering what she had done wrong, the teacher said: 'You are much too fat.' Shelley had no idea what to say. 'You need to go to matron,' she was told, 'and she'll slim you down.' When she arrived in the little office of the school nurse, she explained why she had been sent there. The matron told her to take off all her clothes so she could be examined. As she gazed over Shelley's naked body, she said: 'You're going to die an early death.' The nurse told Shelley she must stop eating in the way that she had been. She gave her no advice about how to achieve that. To the nurse, it was obvious: curtail your greed and laziness.

'I felt so humiliated,' Shelley said. 'It was all shame. It was all shame.' When she heard she was going to die, 'of course, I was terrified'.

She was the only fat girl in the school, and from all directions she constantly received the message that she was disgusting. The other girls would screw up their faces as she walked by and say: 'Oh, you're so fat. I'd hate to be as fat as you.' Shelley told me: 'There were no holds barred. Nobody thought – "Well, that might be hurting her." It was fun for them … The thing about being overweight is that nobody holds back … There's no barriers to stop people.' One day, when she was eating in the school canteen, a teacher said to her: 'I've been watching you, and you're a greedy little girl.' To punish her, she ordered her to eat an extra pudding, then another, then another, like she was a pig at a trough, until finally Shelley vomited.

She internalised everything she was told. She believed she really was disgusting. 'Oh, I hated my body. I couldn't look at myself.' She thought she deserved to be treated this way, and kept thinking: 'I should get thin, and then I'd be a human being, a proper human being.'

Another time, all the girls in her class were lined up to be measured for their gym uniform. The teacher put a tape measure around her and said mockingly, in front of everyone: 'Oh, you're a big girl, aren't you?' As the teacher moved on to the other kids, Shelley turned to the girl next to her and said, distraught: 'I'm fat and I'm ugly and I don't know what to do.' The girl 'looked at me and I could see that she was trying to find something nice to say. She said: "But you've got nice feet."'

Shelley was growing up in Port Talbot, a working-class town in Wales with the largest steelworks in Britain. Her parents were extremely busy running the family pub. As she got home from school, they were getting the bar ready, so they were physically present, but they were never really available. She felt incredibly lonely. Looking back, she realised that her loneliness manifested as a raging hunger for food. She told her mother she felt deeply alone, and out of guilt, her mother offered her food in place of attention. 'She'd leave four doughnuts in a paper bag. I'd come home from school, and there were my doughnuts. They were everything to me.'

In desperation, she tried to diet. It was the late 1960s, and 'what every girl wanted was to be like Twiggy', the famously thin model. 'Everyone was hungry. I mean, really hungry.' To do that, 'you had to starve … People were fainting all over the place.' She tried things like the Grapefruit Diet, where you ate nothing else for days on end. 'I got down to size 16 just once – I think it lasted a day. I've got a photograph of it.' Whenever she couldn't take it any more and broke down, she'd 'eat everything'. Her mother took her to a doctor, who gave her amphetamine-based diet drugs, but 'I didn't feel terribly well on them.' They made her 'heart pound – they affected the rhythm'.

She threw herself into playing music. She was so gifted at playing Bach at the age of thirteen that there were news reports about her. But at school, she reshaped her character in order to get by. 'The only way I could get any kind of belonging to the gang was to be terribly naughty,' she remembered, climbing on desks, throwing things, the thrill of transgression. 'There's the clown,' people would say. As a result, 'I was always in detention.'

Nonetheless, her teachers told her that she was academically gifted and should apply to Cambridge. She couldn't bring herself to do it. She did apply to a different university and was offered a place to study English and psychology – a life-changing offer for a working-class Welsh girl at that time. Her parents were thrilled. But the night before she was supposed to leave, she felt sick with doubt. 'I thought, no, I can't go. I can't go. No. I can't do it. But I wanted to, I really wanted to … I just thought, they'll all be slim, and they'll have a go at me, and I can't cope with it any more.' She never showed up.

Her future seemed like a black hole. She was convinced that she would never get a job and that no man would ever want her. She said to her mother: 'I'm fat and I'm ugly and nobody will ever want anything to do with me … Nobody's going to marry me, but I want babies.' She told me: 'It really worried me. It kept me awake at night, that I wanted these babies, but I can't because I'm too fat.' Then, one day, a skinny man with a sweet smile came into her parents' pub. His name was Alistair. Not long after, he took her on a trip to London, and when he took hold of her hand, 'I thought I was going to die of happiness.' He never once criticised her body. He adored her, and they got married. 'He was very shy, and he was a very good match.'

When she got pregnant with her first child and she went to see the nurse, the first thing she was told was: 'Oh, you shouldn't be having a baby – not at your weight.' Later, as she was lying in the labour ward completely exhausted after a long and difficult birth, the midwife looked at Shelley with contempt and told her she really needed to lose weight. When her son was a year old, she was worried because he wouldn't eat, so she took him to the doctor. He said: 'What are you trying to do? Make the child as fat as yourself?'

Soaking up this abuse all the time was unbearable. As a result, she felt 'I wasn't a proper human being. I didn't belong ... You're not really a person – you're just a body, and it's a bad one.'

~

This kind of cruelty towards overweight people is very widespread. Around 5 per cent of overweight men and 10 per cent of overweight women are insulted or discriminated against every day. For people with a BMI higher than 35, it's much worse – 28 per cent of those men and 45 per cent of the women are soaking up daily abuse. Landlords are 50 per cent less likely to rent their property to a fat person with the same qualifications.

Incredibly, fat people are more likely to be convicted of a crime by juries than slim people.

Some of this shaming is deliberate sadism – but some of it is fear. We often stigmatise the things we are afraid of in ourselves. When *Esquire* magazine polled a thousand women, asking them if they would rather gain 150 pounds or get hit by a truck, more than half of them said they'd prefer the truck. Shelley noticed that the people who were most hostile to her were those who feared gaining weight themselves. She worked for a year with a radio producer who was constantly commenting on her body, and one day the woman said to her: 'You wouldn't believe it, but if I weren't careful all the time, I could end up looking like you.' A friend told Shelley: 'Every time she sees you, she is made aware of what she could become.'

But some of this shaming has a different motive. Many people I have discussed it with seem to sincerely believe that the tool used against Shelley – stigma – is the best way to reduce obesity. Presumably her teacher, and the school nurse, and the midwife, and the doctor, believed that by communicating their disgust at her weight to her, they would push her into shedding it. There is a broadly held belief that stigmatising fat people is for their own good – that it pushes them towards sorting out their health.

So how well does stigma work in reducing obesity? One study of ninety-three women split them into two groups – women who believed they were overweight, and women who didn't. They were all then shown a newspaper article about stigma in the job market towards overweight people. Afterwards, they were all monitored, to see if it had any effect on their eating. It turned out that hearing these claims had no effect on the normal-weight women, but made the women who believed they were overweight eat significantly more. In a different study, overweight people who were shown a harsh and judgemental video ate three times more calories than overweight people who watched a non-judgemental one. There is now a broad range of evidence showing that stigmatising overweight people is in fact counterproductive – on average, it makes them *gain* weight.

There are several reasons for this. The first is fairly obvious. As I learned earlier, if you increase stress, you increase comfort eating. Shelley told me that when she was insulted and degraded for her weight, 'I said to myself – I'm not a real person. And then I thought – I'll go and have something to eat, just this once, just to calm me down.'

Stigma also makes overweight people far less likely to exercise. The Fat Pride activist and bestselling author Aubrey Gordon has written about how, when she was a child, she loved to swim. But then, when she went through puberty, she was made to feel self-conscious whenever she wore a swimsuit, so she stopped. This is really dangerous, because even though exercise doesn't usually cause much weight loss, it hugely boosts your health, whatever size you are. Stigma deters people from seeking out medical help as well: 45 per cent of American women have postponed going to the doctor until they lose weight. Stigma also makes it harder for overweight people to hear necessary medical advice. If you spend your life soaking up abuse about your weight, it's easy to hear well-meant guidance as yet more cruelty.

And there is a deeper reason still. I first heard it articulated by the author Lindy West. She wrote: 'Loving yourself is not antithetical to health, it is intrinsic to health. You can't take good care of a thing you hate.' Shelley said that after all those formative years of being told her body was vile, 'I will tell you something which I've never told anyone before, but I think it's important. I have never seen myself with no clothes on. I absolutely couldn't bear it.' She screwed her eyes shut. Even in the shower, she said, she would look away from her own flesh, appalled by it. How could she learn to look after a body she could not even bear to look at? Why do we believe that making people loathe their bodies will make them take care of them?

~

In the late 1980s, Shelley was working as a journalist, and she realised that nobody in Britain had ever written a book arguing against this cruelty. So, sitting at her desk in her home, she started to do it, not knowing where it would take her. She wrote: 'There is no way to hide being fat except by staying indoors, and so most fat women exist within a tense and stressful straitjacket, unable to be freely themselves, circumscribed by social censure, aware every day in everything they do that they are being defined by their body size.'

She argued that this prejudice – which she had faced almost every day of her life – was cruel, unjust and counterproductive. She began to see it as akin to racism and sexism. She was especially outraged when she read evidence that showed how cruel some doctors could be to fat people. One doctor, named Cecil Webb-Johnson, had written years before: 'A fat man is a joke, and a fat woman is two jokes – one on herself and one on her husband.' She also read testimonies from women that said: 'My doctor said if he had a dollar for every pound I was overweight he could pay off his mortgage'; 'My doctor said I might as well buy a gun and shoot myself'; 'My doctor said I couldn't get pregnant, I was fat, who would want to make me pregnant (and it turned out I was pregnant).'

Shelley thought: What if I stopped being angry with myself, and started being angry with the people insulting me? She learned that in 1969 in the United States, a movement had been formed that called itself Fat Acceptance, later renamed Fat Pride, and they published a manifesto saying: 'We repudiate the mystified "science" which falsely claims that we are unfit.' Shelley called her book *The Forbidden Body*, because that's how it felt: that she was living in a body that was forbidden. It came out in 1989, and that's when, as a little boy, I saw her being mocked on television. People were extremely hostile to her. She was presented as a mad person, promoting sickness and dysfunction. But her bold step was the birth of something in Britain – one of the first times a person had named this stigma, and fought publicly against it. The book became a bestseller, and it was widely discussed. For a while, she was notorious.

~

In the years following Shelley's book and work by other thinkers, Fat Pride activists developed a more detailed set of arguments that eventually went well beyond a simple debunking of stigma. They argued that the entire science of obesity, as presented by the world's doctors and scientists, had been built on a series of errors.

I read their arguments carefully, and it seemed to me they put forward five central factual claims.

Firstly, they argue that many obese people are healthy, and in fact there is growing evidence that it is possible to be 'healthy at any size'.

Secondly, they argue that the science of obesity is based on a basic error. They said it is true that for many people, obesity *correlates* with all sorts of health problems – that if you become more obese, you are more likely to become diabetic, for example. But they say that is not proof that obesity *causes* those problems. The fact that two things happen at the same time is not proof that one causes the other. For example, if you look at the statistics, when sales of ice cream go up, violent crime often goes up too. It would be easy to look at this and assume that ice cream makes people violent. But that's obviously not the case. In fact, what is happening is that a third factor is driving up both violent crime and ice-cream sales – hot weather. The Fat Pride activists argue that similarly, there may be underlying third factors that cause *both* obesity *and* the other health problems. The other factors they warn about include anti-fat stigma, poverty and an obsession with dieting, all of which flood your body with stress, screw with your system and make you sick.

Thirdly, they argue that there is simply a natural variation in human body shapes, based mostly on our genes, and that instead of waging war on that variety, we should help people to find self-acceptance.

Fourthly, they claim that the science of obesity is less certain than it appears to be, since the primary measure used by doctors and scientists, body mass index, is fatally flawed on several fronts. It cannot distinguish between people who have a high muscle mass and those with a high fat mass – a jacked

NFL player will have a similar BMI to a person eating ten KFC buckets a day. Worse still, it is racist: it was designed by a white man in the nineteenth century who used white bodies as his sole measure, ignoring that other ethnic groups can have different body shapes.

Lastly, they also argue that the science was dealt a further blow, starting in 1999. Katherine Flegal is a senior epidemiologist at the Centers for Disease Control and had been one of the first people to warn that obesity had begun to rise dramatically in the US in the early 1980s. She published a study where she and her colleagues had analysed a dataset of over 36,000 people and found something they believed was striking: people who were overweight were slightly *less* likely to die than people of normal weight. This – along with a small number of other seemingly anomalous findings – has been dubbed the 'obesity paradox'.

Shelley was persuaded by some of these arguments. 'I had read a great deal of scientific research that claimed the stated health risks of being overweight were at best exaggerated, at worst simply not true. This was a dastardly ploy by the fat-hating medical profession to rid the world of the dreaded obese.'

~

But Shelley had another problem, one that was starting to make her feel divided in her own mind. By this time, she weighed nineteen and a half stone (273 pounds) and had a BMI above 40, and she was finding that 'physically, it's uncomfortable. You've got a lot of stomachs, and it's heavy to carry around.' She went with her family for a weekend at a theme park named Center Parcs, and she realised she just couldn't walk any significant distance. Her family borrowed a wheelchair, but her husband, who was physically fit, struggled to push her, while her daughter, a fitness instructor, couldn't get her up a slope and had to be helped by strangers. 'I could not help feeling a burden, literally.'

Shelley was also told by her doctor that her heart was strained. She was becoming very worried about her health, and finding it harder and harder to walk. She was only in her fifties.

But she felt that if she talked about this candidly, she would be letting down all the women who looked to her for a celebration of being larger. It became a huge dilemma. She wanted to embrace body positivity, but she wanted to have a healthy body too, and she suspected that obesity was getting in the way of that. Was this a contradiction? How could she reconcile them?

Within the movement, some tensions had already begun to open up. The British Fat Pride movement had a newsletter named *Fat News*, and when a group of women had wanted to write about the challenges of being diabetic in it, they were told they couldn't, because that would present a negative image of being overweight, and the movement was all about showing a positive picture. The only negative aspects that could be acknowledged were discrimination and stigma.

Shelley was very proud of her work opposing stigma, and she would never step back from it. But she felt the movement had to find a way to distinguish between two things – the social harms caused by stigma, and the physical harms caused by being overweight, which would continue to exist to some degree even if there was no stigma in the world. But how could she do that?

~

She started to look at some of the claims made by her allies that obesity is not bad for you, to see if they were true. She wanted to believe them. I also analysed them in great detail, talking them over with some of the most distinguished scientists in the field. (What follows is my understanding, not Shelley's, until I pick up her story again.)

Walter Willett is professor of epidemiology and nutrition at Harvard School of Public Health and Harvard Medical School, and one of the most cited researchers on nutrition in the world. Looking at the first claim – that many obese people are healthy – he told me: 'Nothing is 100 per cent. Not every smoker gets lung cancer, but it dramatically increases your risk.' In a similar way, of course there are some obese people who, even as they age, remain physically fit and free of illness, but sadly, the odds are rigged against them. Obesity 'increases your risk of a broad range of diseases'. He explained that beyond a certain point, the more obese a person becomes, the greater the risk to their health, just as the more a person smokes, the greater their chances of getting lung cancer. So to claim you can reliably be healthy at any size is built on 'a huge amount of denial, and misleading'. He said: 'The tobacco industry used to say, "My grandmother lived to ninety-five, and she was a smoker all her life."' Most people can see why this is misleading. The existence of outliers doesn't disprove statistical risks.

Against this, Fat Pride activists point to a small body of scientific research based on a concept called 'Health at Every Size'. For example, in an experiment run by Dr Lindo Bacon investigating these principles, the scientists involved took a group of overweight women who had tried dieting many times, and split them into two groups. The first tried to count and restrict their calories, in a way that we're all familiar with. The second were offered a different approach. This group would meet every week with a supportive coach, and they would be told, in effect: Stop fixating on your weight. Forget that goal. Focus on something different. Instead, resolve that you are going to live your best life. You are going to eat healthy food. You will exercise. You are going to try and come up with other ways to reward yourself for feeling good than eating ice cream or trying to starve yourself. Stop thinking about your weight, and start thinking about your health. In effect, they were offered Weight Watchers without the focus on weight – a supportive group dedicated to helping them become healthier.

At the end of the experiment, the two groups were compared, and then Lindo went back to them two years later and compared them again. The dieting group lost a small amount of weight, while the second Health at Every Size group did not. But there's a catch. Forty-one per cent of the dieting group dropped out within six months, and even the ones who stuck at it regained a lot of the weight they'd lost, and their self-esteem fell. In comparison, almost nobody dropped out of the Health at Every Size group. They began to eat a little more healthily, increased the amount of time they spent in physical activity, and had higher self-esteem, and these improvements lasted for at least two years. There have now been a few more studies of this approach, and they broadly find the same thing.

Based on these experiments, I think it's reasonable to say that for people who are already overweight and who don't want to take the new weight-loss drugs, there are some real benefits to *emphasising* health at any size – to choosing health as your goal, not necessarily weight loss. But that's very different from saying you *are* healthy at any size, and implying that there is no increased risk from obesity.

Unfortunately the second message is what a lot of people are hearing. For example, Igor Sapozhnikov, a doctor in Panorama City, a working-class neighbourhood in Los Angeles, told me that he has noticed a disturbing shift. Now, when he tries to talk with obese patients about the risks to their health, they increasingly tell him they are healthy and it's wrong to tell them that their weight can affect their health. 'This has been a real challenge,' he said. When he tries to explain the evidence that, over time, obesity hugely increases the chances of diabetes or knee problems, often they push back using arguments based on a distorted understanding of Health at Every Size. 'I just had a patient the other day tell me: "It doesn't matter what my BMI is, because health is individualised." This person has a BMI of 40, which is very high. It's shocking to hear that, because when someone has that BMI, it's almost like pulling a shade over your eyes.' He said that these ideas, and some aspects of Fat Pride, are like 'a false prophet'. They can make you feel good in the short term, but if they make you ignore the long-term risks, you can end up 'having your leg amputated because of diabetes, or [with] such severe arthritis that you can't move and you're stuck in your house. I think tolerance is important in society, and I would be the first person to say that. Absolutely. But I think people are getting the wrong impression of this movement.'

On the second claim – that obesity doesn't cause the broad range of health problems attributed to it, it merely correlates with them – Walter Willett told me that we know obesity causes these problems for many reasons. When you reduce obesity – which he acknowledges is very hard – these problems are massively reduced. Look, he said, at 'the massive changes we get with weight reduction'. I mentioned these statistics earlier but I think they are worth repeating: when people have bariatric surgery, 75 per cent of the people with diabetes see it go away completely, 60 per cent of people with hypertension are cured of it, your chance of dying of cancer falls by 60 per cent, and your chances of being killed by heart disease fall by 56 per cent over five years. Similarly, the weight loss caused by Ozempic reduces strokes and heart attacks by 20 per cent within five years.

How could that be, if some other factor was really causing the problem? Bariatric surgery reverses obesity and only obesity. Ozempic reverses obesity and only obesity. They don't reverse poverty or the other third factors that activists claim could be causing these problems. Yet the evidence shows it dramatically improves your health. 'Stress likely does add to the issue' of the negative effects caused by obesity, Walter said, but 'these are much more powerful changes than have ever been documented by changes in stress'.

There are important truths in the third claim – that human body shapes vary naturally, mostly due to our genes, and it's better to encourage people to accept and love their bodies than to change them. Human body shapes do vary in part because of our genetics. That has always been the case, and always will be. It's always healthier for people to love their bodies than to hate them.

But when I heard some activists say that almost all the variation in weight is determined by genes, I kept reflecting on what I had been taught earlier by scientists about the extraordinary rise in obesity in my lifetime. I thought a lot about an analogy. The weather has always varied based on natural factors, and it always will. But now, as a result of the climate crisis, we are experiencing far more severe heat, and wildfires, and floods, because these natural differences have been supercharged by something else – our greenhouse gas emissions. In the same way, the science I had read showed me there had always been natural variation in our body shapes, but now the extremes have been supercharged. The gap between the thinnest and fattest people more than doubled over the course of the twentieth century. With both the climate and our body shapes, the underlying natural factors have interacted with unnatural factors to produce a risky outcome.

Obviously, the genetic make-up of the human race did not spontaneously transform to make us so much more obese in my lifetime. If weight is fixed entirely or primarily by genes, why has it changed so much, so quickly? To deny the role of genes is absurd; but to deny that your genes interact with the environment to produce your weight is equally absurd. We certainly want self-acceptance. But isn't there a difference between self-acceptance and accepting the effects of a predatory food industry that's poisoned us?

On the fourth claim – that BMI is a bad measure that tells us nothing about health – Walter said: 'BMI is definitely not a perfect measure conceptually because it doesn't separate fat mass from lean mass, [and] that's the fundamental limitation of BMI.' But most people presenting at a doctor's office with high BMIs are not super-muscled, and if they are, the doctor can tell straight away. Walter explained that when it comes to predicting the harms of obesity, BMI 'works amazingly well'. If a doctor measures your BMI and finds it to be over 30, there is 'an extremely high probability' that you also have high excess body fat – which has been proven to have all sorts of negative health effects. Doctors can move to other measures of obesity if they want. For example, they could measure levels of visceral fat, or use something called the body adiposity index, or your waist circumference. All of these can distinguish fat mass from muscle mass, and none of them were invented by nineteenth-century racists, as BMI undoubtedly was. Yet Walter stressed that the scientific evidence shows they match up pretty closely with BMI, and when you use them you find very similar negative outcomes from being overweight.

The final claim is the most complex, and it took me a while to grasp it. If you look at any graph of how your body weight affects your chances of dying, it will always have a familiar shape. Picture a curve in the shape of the letter U. At the left-hand side of the U, where people are very thin, there is a high risk of dying. Then as people become a more normal weight, the chance of dying drops, and there's a fairly long and gentle curve. Then at the right-hand side of the U, where people get too overweight, the risk of dying shoots up again. Everyone who works on obesity science agrees that this U exists, and that it accurately describes the connection between weight and death.

But as I mentioned before, in 1999, Katherine Flegal noticed something odd when she was studying the data behind this U-curve. She found that in the US, it is indeed dangerous to be too thin or too overweight, but the group who seemed to be least likely to die were in fact people who are slightly overweight, with a BMI between 25 and 29. They made up the lowest dip in the U. This bolstered the argument that there is an 'obesity paradox'. Fat Pride activists often use her research to argue that being fat isn't actually as bad for you as we keep being told.

Walter told me that this argument is based on a mistake. Katherine Flegal had looked at the raw death rates for large numbers of people across the whole spectrum of BMIs, from thin to obese. But, he said, if you want to know the effects of obesity on people's health, this isn't a good idea – because those figures are polluted by two other big factors that skew the results. Heavy smokers are significantly more likely to be in the 'non-obese' category, because nicotine is an appetite suppressant, but it also kills you sooner. At the same time, seriously ill and dying people are more likely to be in the 'non-obese' category, because when you are sick or dying, you usually lose weight. These factors, in combination, mean that her data gives a 'misleading answer'. If you want to know what obesity does to you, he said, you need to compare people with a healthy weight who don't smoke and aren't dying, to obese people who don't smoke and aren't dying. He said he has done that many times in his research, and it always shows there is 'pretty much a straight line relationship between body weight and mortality'. Above a BMI of 25, your risk of dying starts to rise. So 'there is no obesity paradox', he said, and the idea that there is one is 'disconnected from the realities of biology'.

In response to this critique, Katherine Flegal then did another large-scale study, where she worked very hard to exclude smokers and people who were dying from her data. She still found that slightly overweight people were the least likely to die. When Walter read her new analysis, he argued that her published data did *not* properly exclude those groups, and therefore was still polluted. A complex and quite bitter argument over this is still ongoing, with serious scientists on both sides. But in the many years since Katherine Flegal's unexpected findings were first published, no major medical body in the world has changed its advice and said that it's good for your health to have a BMI of between 25 and 29. The other evidence is just too strong.

When I read all these studies, the most important fact that struck me is that both Walter and Katherine and all the scientists in the field agree that beyond a BMI of 30, your risk of dying starts to rise, and it rises really substantially above 35. They agree on the overall shape of the U-curve. In the end, Katherine's findings, sadly, don't bolster the Fat Pride case in the way they seem to think it does.

~

Shelley told me in a level voice: 'I've looked at the science, and it can't be said that it won't harm you' to be obese. She believes 'we have to deal in reality'.

She wanted these claims that obesity doesn't harm you to be true, but she could feel in her body – and see in the data – that they were not. She wrote: 'The truth is that beyond a certain weight' our bodies 'let us down. It is futile to protest that this is not so. I believe in dealing in reality … Being fat is never a sin. It's never anybody's fault. But it can be disabling in many senses and I believe it's essential that we don't deny or gloss over that.' She also emphasised: 'That there are health problems at high weights is irrefutable; to deny this would be burying our heads in the sand.'

When she was young, Shelley was obese and fairly healthy, just like most smokers in their twenties have healthy lungs; but by middle age, the risks were catching up with her. A study by scientists at University College London followed a group of 2,521 British government bureaucrats – whose weights ranged broadly – over twenty years, to track their health. At the start, a third of the obese people in the study were healthy. But then, as the years passed, a majority of the healthy obese people became unwell, and after they crunched the statistics, the scientists concluded that obesity made you eight times more likely to become unwell.

So where did this leave Shelley? People told her: 'You can't lose weight – you'd be betraying the cause.' She replied: 'What do they mean? What is the cause? To me, it's about the solidarity of fat people against a hostile society ... It doesn't mean maintaining a high weight.'

She decided to go to a weight-loss support group near where she lived. This wasn't easy – she had been very critical of these groups in her book, comparing them to fundamentalist churches, and saying that they nurtured self-hate. But when she went in, 'I thought, I'm going to set aside everything I know about fatness and thinness and eating and all that, and just be part of this particular group.' They explained that you were given a little book where you had a range of healthy fresh food options you prepared yourself, and every day, you had to choose three of them. Then every week, you'd meet, talk about it, and weigh yourself. It 'seemed to me to be just sensible – ordinary women, with an ordinary way of doing it'.

In the first week, she said, 'I don't think I've lost anything,' and the woman leading the group said, 'Come on the scales, we'll see.' She had lost half a stone. To her surprise, as time went on, 'actually, it worked'. She lost seven stone in a year, and she kept it off successfully for eighteen years. Then she had an emotionally devastating experience in her family, and gained two stone, where she has remained ever since. Previously, she had quoted an American researcher who said that 'to expect a fat person to become thin is as unreasonable as expecting a Black person to bleach her skin or a Jew to convert to Christianity'. But now, although Shelley was not thin, she had dramatically reduced her weight. She knew she was part of a minority for whom changing how you eat worked in the long term, and she was humble about that. But she felt much better in her body, her health was recovering, and she wanted to tell the truth about it.

~

One day she was visiting Edinburgh, and she saw a bus she wanted stopping on Princes Street. She knew that if she ran, she could catch it. As she boarded, she felt breathless and exhilarated.

She had gone from almost losing her ability to walk, to being able to run. She said she couldn't deny there was a difference. Being able to run was better.

~

Shelley has come to believe that we can – and must – reconcile two important goals. We need to reduce the stigma that harms people's minds, and at the same time, wherever possible, we need to reduce the excess weight that harms people's bodies. They are both forces that hurt people, and we can move towards dismantling both with love and compassion. There is, she says, no contradiction between these twinned goals.

But to some people in the movement, she has been seen as a traitor for saying this. Shelley regards these people with sympathy. She believes they are 'too frightened' to acknowledge the reality. 'I think there's so much fear in this. Different kinds of fear ... There's so much denial.' It's not hard to see why. If you spend your life soaking up abuse, it's very easy to hear even well-meant and well-sourced concern about your health as yet more abuse. If the only tool that you've ever heard to promote change is shame, then of course you're going to be resistant to these ideas. There's another reason why it's so difficult for some people. As I discussed before, overeating performs all sorts of positive psychological functions for many of us: it soothes us, it re-enacts deep childhood patterns, it keeps us safe from most sexual predators. When somebody talks about the risks of obesity, what many people hear is: You're threatening to take away the thing that makes me safe.

As a result of some combinations of these motives, many of her former friends lashed out at Shelley, arguing that she had given in to stigma and was now just repeating the false things that are said about fat people. Yet she believes that she would be dead now if, all those years ago, she hadn't truly absorbed the science of what obesity can do to your body and found a way to change. She began to wonder: what kind of body positivity is it that would shame her for keeping her body alive? How can you be positive about your body if it ceases to exist? 'I don't know how you get around that,' she said, with a shake of her head.

As she said this, I thought about how Ozempic and the other new weight-loss drugs are going to reshape the debate on body positivity. A polarised debate is taking shape here. Because they have spent years claiming that obesity doesn't harm your health, some of the Fat Pride activists can only make sense of these drugs as weapons of prejudice. One famous figure in the movement, for example, the writer Aubrey Gordon – who has made good points in other contexts – said in an interview that the primary driving force behind Ozempic was to say: 'Can we finally be rid of fat people? … Can we finally stop having fat people around, so I don't have to look at them any more?'

But soon, almost all obese people will know somebody who is going to take these drugs, lose a huge amount of weight, and see all sorts of huge benefits for their health and their quality of life. I thought again of Jeff Parker, the retired lighting designer I interviewed, who is now enjoying his retirement and walking his little dog over the Golden Gate Bridge, after receiving test results showing his health problems are vanishing. Most people who take these weight-loss drugs then become advertisements for them, revealing that you can lose weight relatively painlessly, and significantly boost your health. It was never scientifically plausible to deny that obesity caused these problems, but as this happens, it will also become emotionally less plausible too.

I want to make sure that when that takes place, we don't see a collapse of the body positivity movement. We need a movement that opposes stigma against overweight people: it's cruel, it's destructive and it makes the problem worse. It degrades and wounds people. Even if we are able to return to the range of human body shapes we used to have before processed food super-sized us, there will still be a lot of variation and variety. We need a movement that says that it's neither possible nor desirable for all of us to aim to look like Kate Moss or Timothée Chalamet; that builds your self-esteem on more than your waist size; that asserts the moral worth and dignity of every human being, and stands up to bullying. If the movement is tied to denying that obesity can harm human health, then it is unlikely to survive except as a very marginal force. If it is tied to these wider moral truths – ones Shelley has played a role in articulating since the 1980s – then it will be as needed as ever.

Shelley believes there is a sensible middle ground here. 'There are many large women – I would say the majority – who have a passionate commitment to bringing about an end of prejudice, and yet are not happy or comfortable in their own bodies,' she wrote. As a result, 'we have to find a way of reconciling size acceptance and weight loss'.

We have two tasks ahead of us – to learn to love our bodies however they are, and to learn to make our bodies as healthy and functional as we can. There is no contradiction between the two, because both are forms of self-love. She believes that 'things are never either/or. They are both/and.' In a radically simplifying age driven by social media rage, it's hard to present the case for complexity and compassion, but she is determined to do it.

~

After our long day talking, Shelley's husband Alistair came to collect her from the pub in his car. As they walked across the car park, he took her hand, like he had on a day trip to London nearly fifty years before, filling her with joy. While I watched her go, I realised that she had pioneered a brave and necessary way of taking on stigma in the 1980s – and she may also have pioneered the more complex way we are going to have to think about body positivity now in the age of potentially radical weight loss. Not either/or. Both/and.

12

The Land That Doesn't Need Ozempic

What the Japanese do right – and how we can become like them

In July 2023, I stumbled across a curious news story. It appeared in the Pharma Letter, a media outlet that covers the pharmaceutical industry for people who work in it and for investors. It explained what sounds, at first glance, like good news for Novo Nordisk, the company that makes Ozempic and Wegovy. The drug had just been approved to treat obesity in Japan. That surely would mean a bonanza: the country has the third largest economy in the world, and a population of over 125 million people.

But here's where the article turned sober. A market analyst interviewed by the site predicted that while these drugs would come to dominate the market for anti-obesity medicines in Japan, that doesn't mean much, because there is almost no obesity there. Just 4.5 per cent of its people are obese, compared to 26 per cent of people in the UK, and 42.5 per cent in the US. Even more strikingly, the report said that obesity in the country is projected to shrink by 0.8 per cent a year. As a result, the market for these drugs will, the article noted, be 'slow'.

This is part of a bigger picture – one I kept getting tantalising hints of throughout my research for this book. Japan is the only country in the world that got rich without getting fat. It's strange that sumo wrestlers are one of the most recognisable symbols of the country, because expecting other Japanese people to look like them is like expecting Americans to look like a bald eagle.

Naturally, when I read this news story, I wanted to understand: how did Japan become the land that doesn't need Ozempic? If we want to avoid a future where we are forced to choose between widespread obesity and weight-loss drugs, might it hold the key?

~

My first assumption was that the Japanese must have won the genetic lottery – there had to be something in their DNA that makes them stay so slim. When I began to dig into this question, I learned that something happened over a hundred years ago that has helped scientists to figure out if it was true.

In the late nineteenth and early twentieth century, large numbers of Japanese workers migrated to Hawaii and they have now been living on the islands for four generations. They are genetically very similar to the Japanese people who didn't leave, but living in a very different environment. So by looking at these different groups, scientists were able to investigate: is Japanese people's slimness indelibly written into their genes, or does it change when the environment changes?

It turns out that after a hundred or so years, Japanese-Hawaiians are now almost as fat as the people they live among. Some 17 per cent of them are obese, compared to 25 per cent of Hawaiians of other ethnic groups. Japanese-Hawaiians are more than four times more likely to be obese than people back in Japan. The fact that their obesity level is slightly lower than other Hawaiian groups suggests Japanese people's genes may make them a bit less likely to gain weight – but only a bit. Clearly something else is going on. But what?

~

The only way to find out was to go to Japan, and as soon as I thought about this, I knew there was one person I wanted to take with me. Six years before, I had gone on a disastrous holiday with my teenage godson Adam, which I wrote about in my book *Stolen Focus: Why You Can't Pay Attention.* (I have changed his name and a few minor identifying details.) He was spending all his time staring at Snapchat and YouTube, and his ability to pay attention had shattered into tiny Snapchat-sized fragments. To try to break this numbing routine, I took him on a road trip all over the American South. Before we left, he promised he would leave his phone in the hotel during the day – but he couldn't do it. He constantly stared at his screen, and we ended up screaming at each other in Graceland, shouting at each other outside the White House, and shrieking at each other on the Bayou.

But by the time I decided to go to Japan, he was a transformed man. He had found a job he loved, helping people with addiction problems, and a girlfriend he really liked, and slowly, he had built up a life where he wanted to be present and pay attention. This had led him to make another change. When he hit his teens, he had rapidly gained weight, and by his early twenties, he weighed twenty stone (280 pounds). But the same factors that had made it possible for him to slash back his social media use seemed to also make it possible for him to lose a huge amount of weight. Now that he had a life he wanted to live for, he had lost eight stone (112 pounds), mostly by dramatically cutting back on junk food. People he had known for years would walk past him in the street because they didn't recognise him.

It was joyful to see him no longer wheezing and feeling sick if he had to walk even short distances, and now looking so confident and full of health. But at the back of my mind, I kept worrying about those statistics I had learned, showing that 80 per cent of people who lose weight on diets regain it over the next few years. I wondered if seeing whatever magic they had uncovered in Japan might help him to stay healthy. This time, I didn't even need to ask him to leave his phone in the hotel: he hardly looked at it these days.

~

So in late August, in an intense summer heat wave, we touched down in Tokyo. On the first morning, in our hotel, I noticed there were two breakfasts laid out side by side. To the right, there was the breakfast for Japanese guests. It consisted of small pieces of fresh grilled fish, some pickles and tiny bowls of soup. To the left, there was the breakfast for Western guests. It consisted of scrambled eggs, French fries, piles of bacon, pancakes and lots of buttered toast.

I decided that to learn about the Japanese diet, I should live on it for the sixteen days we were there. I was sitting at the table sipping soup when Adam returned from the buffet. 'I just saw the weirdest thing,' he said in an elevated whisper. 'A Japanese woman had taken some fish and some pickles from their part of the buffet. Then she walked over to where our food was, picked up the prongs, and took a single chip, and put it on her plate. Then she put it back, and put an even smaller chip on her plate, because she clearly thought the first one was too big.' He nodded discreetly to where she was sitting. I turned and saw the single small French fry, sitting there on her plate, next to the white fish she was slowly chewing.

~

After we finished eating, Adam and I headed straight for the symbolic centre of the city, the Shibuya Crossing – a mad spot where seven roads collide and all the traffic lights go red at the same time, triggering an orderly crush of people crossing in all directions. As we joined the 2.4 million people who hurry across it every day, we glanced up at the enormous electronic screens flashing all around us. I almost froze in shock when I saw a giant three-dimensional image of a dog that seemed to be leaping out of the screen towards us. For a British person of my generation, it's strange to come to Japan for the first time, because when I was a teenager, this is what I thought my own future would look like – a dense, squashed, neon frenzy. But like hoverboards, that alternative world didn't come to pass. I felt like I had arrived in yesterday's future, one that never quite happened.

For lunch, we bought some sushi in a random part of a railway station for four dollars each. I assumed it would be the equivalent of those sweaty sandwiches you get in service stations across the US and Britain, but in fact, it was fresh and delicious. 'This tastes so good,' Adam said, in shock.

To understand why Japanese food is so different, we went to the Tokyo College of Sushi and Washoku to interview

Masaru Watanabe, who is one of the most respected teachers of Japanese cuisine in the country. He had agreed to cook a meal with us and some of his trainees, and to explain the principles behind it. When we arrived, he was waiting by the entrance in an impeccably tailored suit and his socks. (Japanese people don't wear shoes indoors.) He bowed deeply as soon as he saw us and led us into a steel kitchen, where two of his chefs were already at work. 'The Japanese cuisine's [core] feature is simplicity,' Masaru said. 'For us, the simpler, the better. For example – sushi is such a simple food, right? Just a bowl of rice and sliced fish on top. So it's very simple – simple shape, and simple taste. But the simpler [it is], the more difficult' it is to actually prepare, 'because if it's simpler', they have to pay more attention to every detail and make every flavour fire.

He explained that we were going to make a typical Japanese meal, the kind people were eating all over the country that lunchtime. We would grill a mackerel, boil some rice, make some miso soup, and prepare some pickles. You'll notice, he said, that in our meals, we have very small portions, but more of them – five in a typical meal. This means that every Japanese meal contains a much broader range of ingredients. Usually, there are sixty to sixty-five ingredients used, while in a comparable meal cooked in the classic French style, there would be around twenty ingredients. (As he said this, I thought of what Tim Spector had discovered in London – that the more diverse your diet, the healthier your gut, and the more your overall health improves.)

His chefs grilled a mackerel, and I watched as various oils and fats leeched out of it and dripped down. He told me that Japanese people mainly live on fish and vegetables, not milk and butter and meats. 'We don't traditionally eat meat a lot. We are an island country. We appreciate fish.' He pointed to the dripping oils, and said: 'With this process, you reduce the oil and fat of the fish itself, making it much healthier.'

Even more importantly, Masaru explained, this way of grilling the mackerel is an illustration of one of the crucial principles of Japanese cooking. Western cooking, he said, is primarily about 'adding'. To make a food tasty, you add butter, lemon, herbs, sauces. 'But the Japanese style is totally the opposite.' It's 'a minus cuisine'. This cooking is about drawing out the innate flavour, 'not to add anything extra'. The whole point is to try 'to make as much as possible of the ingredients' natural taste'. To them, less is more. On the hob next to us, the rice we were going to eat was slowly cooking in a clay bowl. One of his chefs explained that the clay distributes the heat more evenly, and so draws out more of the natural flavour of the rice.

Another key rule of Japanese cooking, Masaru told me, is that each meal should have 'five tastes, five skills and five colours'. The five tastes – spread across the different small portions – are sweetness, saltiness, sourness, bitterness and umami (which is a kind of savoury taste). They 'try to make these five tastes in combination in one plate', because when you do this, 'the balance of nutrients will be perfect' and it is healthier. The five skills you should aim to use in preparing each meal are cutting, simmering, grilling, deep-frying and steaming. And the five colours you should aim to have on your plate are black, white, green, yellow and red. The blackness often comes from seaweed, which is one of the most popular foods in Japan, and 'has a lot of natural mineral ingredients inside: calcium, potassium', he said. 'It makes your blood pressure lower.'

As the different parts of our meal gradually became ready, his chefs added small edible flowers and tiny Japanese citruses to the side of our plates. By the time they laid the meal in front of us, it looked more like jewellery than a typical American or British meal, because it was so beautiful. He told me that everywhere in Japan, no matter where I went, I would find food presented like this. To them, he said, 'food is a total art, not just a taste art. What you can see is important. Beautiful plating is important. Japanese people really love the details. God lives in the details.'

Before we started to eat, he explained that he would need to teach us how to consume this meal, because if we used normal Western principles of eating, we would get it wrong.

The first thing we had to learn was 'triangle eating'. In the West, he said, if you are given a meal with five different components, you eat them sequentially, one after another – you start the soup, you finish the soup; then you start the salad, and you finish the salad; then you start the pasta, and you finish the pasta. 'In Japan, this is regarded as really weird,' he said. 'It's a rude way of eating.' A meal like this should be eaten in a triangle shape. 'First, drink the soup a little bit, then go to the side dish – one bite. Then try the rice, for one bite. Then the mackerel – again, a single mouthful. Then go back and have another taste of the soup ... This is also the key to keep you healthy ... Keeping the balance, so you don't eat too much.'

The second thing we had to learn is that in Japan, you are meant to combine the different foods in your mouth. Take a bite of the mackerel, chew it a little, and then, before you swallow, add in some of the pickle, or some of the rice, or one of the edible flowers, and chew that too. 'The chef cooks the dishes, but in the end, it is you who does the final cooking in your mouth.' One of his chefs said: 'In that way, Japanese food is something you can enjoy, because you can try out different things and make different flavours.'

The third thing we had to learn is when to stop. In Japan, you are taught from a very early age to only eat until you feel you are 80 per cent full. Eating until you are totally full is regarded as bad for you. It takes time for your body to sense you've had enough, and if you hit a sense of fullness when you are still eating, then you've definitely had too much.

Adam and I started to eat the food in this way – consuming it in a triangle shape, combining it in our mouths, and stopping at 80 per cent. I didn't think adding together a tiny radish and a tiny yellow flower in my mouth could make me so happy, but it felt like a genuinely new flavour-burst I hadn't experienced before.

There was no dessert. When I asked about this, Masaru said: 'We don't have desserts so often. It's for a special occasion. A daily meal?' He shook his head. For a small 'taste of sweetness', they might have some fruit.

He told me that when he was studying, he lived in Ohio for a year and a half, and he was struck that 'they eat much more than I expected. They eat too much – as if they don't have any sense of filling up. They eat *so* much.' He was startled when he heard people say: 'Hey, pasta – it's just a starter. We need meat after the pasta.' When he first saw cheesecake, he was taken aback. As he recalled it, he said with a puckered face: 'I cannot enjoy that.' When he tried eating like an American, he felt terrible. He looked down and said: 'Diarrhoea.' He told me: 'I'm really sorry for them. All that junk food is not good for your health.' In the West, he believes, of 'the recent major diseases for adults, maybe half of them are due to their daily food. Too much salt? Then your blood veins are going to be more stiff, then you get high blood pressure ... Junk food tends to change your body like that.'

Adam told him that in Britain, it's a tradition at Christmas to eat so much that you can't move and you go into a 'food coma'. Masaru's eyes widened. He looked dumbfounded, and didn't know what to say. 'Well,' he said at last, 'it's totally opposite from our culture.'

Discreetly changing the subject, Masaru told me there's another crucial aspect of Japanese cuisine that we should know about. Most Japanese people eat fermented food regularly. One of the most popular foodstuffs is something called natto, which I tried later – it consists of slightly rotten soybeans that have been left to ferment for days. It stinks. Adam wouldn't try it at all. Yet it tasted strangely delicious. Eating this food is important, Masaru said, because it increases good bacteria in your gut.

As we gathered our things and began to leave, I had a nagging worry. Everything we had tasted was delicious and strange – but I didn't feel like I had eaten much. Even with the effects of the Ozempic, I thought I would be hungry soon afterwards. But, strangely, neither I nor Adam was hungry again until that evening. I wondered why, and I thought back to the research I had read earlier, about which foods created a feeling of being sated, and which don't. The Japanese diet is full of foods that create satiety, even in fairly small portions – fish, beans, vegetables.

As we bowed goodbye to Masaru, he nodded towards our empty plates and said: 'When you eat this type of food every day, you're going to be healthy, and live longer.'

~

But I was also conscious that he is a prestigious, high-end chef. I wondered: How widely followed are these principles in everyday life in Japan? I went to a supermarket, and as I walked its aisles, I saw that its shelves and fridges were predominantly lined with fresh fish and fruit and vegetables. I could see very few pre-packaged foods. The whole place was based on the assumption that you were buying ingredients that you would then cook into a meal. There was a small section marked 'Processed Food', with a few tins and packages. In the US and Britain, processed food makes up most of the supermarket. Here, it was a wan and neglected corner.

Three days into eating nothing but Japanese food, I began to experience an odd mixture of hope and humiliation. Often, in the West, people argue that obesity has a simple cause – the sheer amount of food that surrounds us. The argument goes like this: nothing in our evolution prepared us for an ongoing bounty of food. All of our instincts were developed in environments where food was scarce and famine was a constant danger, so when we come across food, our instincts tell us to eat all of it. If we find a lot, we'll eat a lot. So in a rich country with a surplus of food, we will inevitably overeat, and lots of us will become obese. It's a tale that induces despair, or – at best – presents the new weight-loss drugs as the only option. But Japan's experience suggests that there's something wrong with this story. Japan is extraordinarily rich. Everyone in Japan – even the poorest citizens – has access to a surplus of food. Yet they have avoided the obesity trap. It is possible. This is not written into the destiny of every wealthy country.

But as soon as these happy thoughts rushed in, I thought – yes, but the Japanese people have done it in a way we can't possibly replicate. They built up a totally different relationship to food over thousands of years, and we can hardly import that.

So I was surprised to learn that actually most of Japan's current food culture was invented very recently – in living memory, in fact. Barak Kushner, who is professor of East Asian History at Cambridge, has explained that until the 1920s, Japanese cooking was just 'not very good' – fresh fish was eaten only once a week, the diet was dangerously low in protein, and even the techniques of stewing or stir-frying weren't used. Life expectancy was forty-seven. He told the food writer Bee Wilson: 'Japanese culture is neither timeless nor unchanging.' It was only when Japan's imperialist government was creating an army to attack other parts of Asia that they were disturbed that the population ate so badly and was so weak, and a new food culture began to be invented, quite consciously, to produce healthier soldiers. After the defeat of Japan in the Second World War, when the country was in ruins, the new democratic government realised that if they didn't have a healthy population, they would have nothing, and they stepped up this transformation. 'The Japanese only really started eating what we think of as Japanese food in the years after the Second World War,' Bee says. 'Instead of being dispirited by the way the Japanese eat, we should be encouraged by it. Japan shows the extent to which food habits evolve.'

~

So how did the Japanese create this radically different way of eating? To find out, I arrived at Koenji Gakuen School with my translator on a stiflingly hot September morning. It's a typical school for kids aged from five to eighteen in a middle-class residential neighbourhood in Tokyo, and – like at every Japanese school – the kids stream in every morning after walking to school on their own, without adults. Parents wave their kids goodbye at the front door and send them off for this form of morning exercise, starting when they are around six years old.

We were greeted near the entrance by Harumi Tatebe, a woman in her early fifties, who told us she had been the nutritionist at this school for three years. As we walked through the corridors, kids waved at her affectionately, and shouted her name, eager to know what they were having for lunch that day. By law, Harumi said, every Japanese school has to employ a professional like her. It took her three years to qualify, on top of her teaching degree, and she explained that in this position, you have several important roles to play. You design the school meals, in line with strict rules stipulating that they must be fresh and healthy. You oversee the cooking of the school meals. You use these meals to educate the children about nutrition. Then you educate their parents on the same topic. And finally, you provide support and counselling to any kids who are undereating or overeating. She said: 'I've always loved eating. I enjoy eating, and I like watching people who are eating, and looking happy when they eat!'

We arrived at the kitchen and stared in through a large glass panel. Harumi told me that today's meal consisted of five small portions: some white fish, a bowl of noodles with vegetables, milk, some sticky white rice and a tiny dollop of sweet paste. All the kids eat the same meal, and packed lunches are forbidden. No processed or frozen food ever goes into any of the meals here. Even if they use something as simple as curry paste, they don't buy it pre-made. 'We start from scratch.' I asked her why, and she said: 'It's all about nutrition ... Sometimes with frozen food, they use a lot of artificial additives.'

Once the meal was ready, Harumi carried a tray over to the office of the school's head, Minoru Tanaka. It is customary that the principal has the same lunch as the kids, and he eats it first, to make sure it's safe, nutritious and delicious. He rolled up his sleeves and started to eat. After a moment, he nodded to her that it was good. Once he had given this green light, a group of eight children from each class arrived at the kitchen, dressed in little chef outfits. They collected a trolley and pushed it back to their classroom. The kids dressed as cooks stood at the front of the class while the others stepped forward to be served. (This is as adorable as it sounds.) Before they began to eat, a child then stood at the front of the class and read out what today's meal was, which part of Japan it came from, and how the different elements are good for your health. She then said '*Meshiagare!*', the Japanese equivalent of 'bon appétit', and everyone applauded.

While the kids were eating, Harumi held up four coloured ropes. Each one represented a different kind of food you need to be healthy – on this day, they represented carbohydrates, calcium, carbohydrates containing additional calcium and green vegetables. She held up the yellow rope, representing carbs, and asked what they do for your health. A child yelled: 'Give you energy!' She held up the red rope, representing calcium, and a child shouted out that it makes your bones stronger. As she went through the food groups, she tied each rope together, to show that in combination they make a healthy meal. She told me: 'By eating this school lunch every day, which is well balanced, they learn what a balanced meal is.' The principal, Mr Tanaka, agreed, saying: 'Through the school lunches, we explain the food itself.'

Often, Harumi tells the kids: 'Your body is made up of what you're eating right now. Your body's cells are replenished every three months. So what you're eating makes your body now, and your future body … You have to eat with your brain.'

My translator and I walked from class to class, asking the kids what they most liked to eat. The first child I spoke to, a ten-year-old girl, said: 'I like green vegetables, like broccoli.' The next kid said he liked fish. The third said he loved seaweed rice. I asked why, and he said: 'I don't usually like the seaweed, but if it's cooked with rice, I can eat it,' and he was proud that he'd expanded his palate. One eleven-year-old boy told me he loves rice because 'the rice has protein. If you eat balanced food every meal, then you have a very strong body,' and he flexed his tiny biceps, and giggled.

I asked my translator: Is this a joke? Are they trolling me? A bunch of ten-year-olds, telling me how much they love broccoli, fish, seaweed and rice? But most of the Japanese people I discussed this with were puzzled to see that I was puzzled. We teach kids to enjoy healthy food, they explained. Don't you?

As I walked around, I had a nagging sense that there was something unusual about this place, but it was only after a few hours that I realised what it was. There were no overweight children. None. I asked Harumi if there were any, and she told me there was one kid she was worried about. That's one overweight child, out of nearly a thousand students.

And yet it was clear that this is not a culture that teaches kids to deprive themselves of food. The meal the kids ate was hearty, and filling. 'I think it's important to enjoy eating, and enjoy meals,' Harumi said. 'I never say, "No, you can't have that." If you like cake, you can have that. If you like fried chicken, you can of course have that. But if you have it every day, it might not be very good.' They have a mission to encourage children to expand their tastes, and learn to like new foods that they might not enjoy at first. Some kids, she explained, find the taste of vegetables horrible when they initially try them. So she turns it into a game, asking them to help prepare the vegetables, and then challenging them to try just a little bit of what they have made for themselves. 'I am always impressed by how they grow up,' she said.

As the kids finished up their lunch, I pulled out my phone, and showed them photographs of typical American and British school meals, to see what they made of them. I deliberately didn't choose the most disgusting meals – just images of the normal mixture of fried food, chips and baked beans that I grew up eating from my school canteen. When they saw the pictures, they gasped. 'Oh my God!' one little boy cried out in English. Another yelled: 'It looks disgusting!' One asked incredulously: 'Did you eat like this every day?'

I asked a twelve-year-old girl, who seemed to be stunned into silence, what she was thinking. She tilted her head and said: 'It's very greasy. It might be very strenuous for your body.' Another boy asked: 'Is there no salad with that?' I said that I never ate a salad at school, not a single time. He looked taken aback, and told me: 'It's better if you eat it. It's good for your health. It's good to be healthy. If you don't eat salad, you'll gain weight, or have stomach problems.'

Another child, looking pained, said: 'I think you're missing a lot in life if you don't eat salad.' Then she touched my arm and, clearly trying to find a way to incentivise me to expand my palate, said: 'It goes well with meat.'

~

The next day, in a different school in another part of Tokyo, I showed a group of mothers the same photos. They looked equally stunned. One of them, a woman named Maiko Arai, asked me – is there a movement, to change this terrible situation?

I looked back at her, and didn't know what to say.

~

Up until this point, Adam and I had been seeing aspects of Japan's approach towards health that seemed to me to be totally admirable. But next, I looked at a crucial part of their model that left me with mixed feelings. In 2008, the Japanese government noticed that obesity was slightly rising (although it was still laughably low by our standards). Panicked, they introduced a piece of legislation which became known as the 'Metabo Law', because it was designed to reduce one of the nastiest effects of obesity – metabolic syndrome, a combination of obesity, diabetes and high blood pressure that really trashes your health. The law contained a simple rule. Once a year, every workplace in Japan has to bring in a team of nurses and doctors to measure the weight and waistline of every employee aged between 40 and 75, and if they have gone up, the company and the employee need to draw up a health plan together to bring them back down.

I couldn't imagine how this could possibly work, so I wanted to see it in practice. A company called Tanita agreed to let me talk to their employees about it, and to see the measures they have put in place. They make vegan food, healthy meal replacements and exercise equipment, so they are especially keen to promote a healthy Japan, and for the world to know about it.

When I arrived at their reception, I laughed. In what looked like a parody of how the world views Japan, the first things I saw were a giant seven-foot robot and an image of Hello, Kitty skipping. (The robot, I learned later, was designed by the company with Sega for a video game that promotes exercise.) If you are an employee of Tanita, when you arrive at the office, you check in by standing in front of a large video screen. It scans your face and then greets you with your name and some information about you. Every employee has to wear a device that measures how many steps you walk every day, and it immediately tells you where you are in the company ranking. 'Hello, Bob,' it might say, 'you are 143rd in the ranking of how many steps were taken yesterday.' If you haven't weighed yourself in the past week on one of the office scales, it reminds you to do it, and if any of the colleagues who sit near you have forgotten to, it tells you to remind them that they need to. It congratulates you if you have reached a new milestone. 'Congratulations,' it says, 'you have walked the equivalent of the entire distance of the Tokyo loop line on the subway this year.'

Everyone who works here is encouraged to post a photo of all the meals they eat, and they are then displayed publicly on the video screen, so that everyone can scroll through what their colleagues have been eating. You can also read all your colleagues' commitments to improve their health, with their names next to it. I saw that one man had pledged: 'I will try to drink on average less than once a month.' Another promised: 'I will not have a second serving.' Another: 'I will try to eat balanced meals with a lot more vegetables, and only until I am 80 per cent full.'

Different companies stay in line with the Metabo Law in different ways, and Tanita is at the most enthusiastic edge. But all over Japan, workplaces encourage health in their own way.

As I was led upstairs by Hiro Yokota, Tanita's head of public relations, employees were gathering in the break room for their morning exercises. Like in most Japanese workplaces, every morning at 9 a.m., at a time when in Western offices people are eating doughnuts and chugging coffee, everyone gathers to do some aerobics together. People arrived holding their own giant floppy green elastic band made by the company, and then a perky recorded voice began to blare into the room. It told them what to do. Raise your arms in the air and tilt to your left; now tilt to your right; now lean forward. Everyone followed along, and soon, on command, they were leaping up and down in little star jumps. It was light but not unchallenging, and it was interesting to see the older employees joining in as vigorously as the younger ones. Everyone knew the moves, and there was a jolly atmosphere. It was strangely beautiful to see them all moving in unison, their giant green bands stretched taut.

After around ten minutes, people parted and headed to their desks. In a side office, the first person I met with was Junya Nagasawa, the company's boss. He is a handsome 57-year-old who consistently comes top of the company's walking league table, with nearly 20,000 steps a day. When the Metabo Law came into force, he told me, there was a sudden demand from companies for technologies that could help them to monitor their employees' health and find ways to improve it. So Tanita designed these video screens and health surveillance systems, and he felt that if you're going to sell them, you've got to put your money where your mouth is and apply them in your own workplace. As a result, he started to walk much more. 'I think it is very important to incorporate walking as part of your daily routine,' he said. 'In reality, it's not difficult to walk, but it's very difficult to make the time. Because I'm a businessman, I'm always busy. For me, I try to use my free time before I come to work. That's the only hour I actually have control over.' Now, he gets up earlier, and gets off the subway four stops sooner to walk the rest of the way. 'I had to be the role model,' he said. 'I couldn't have not walked. I lost weight. I felt lighter. I rarely catch a cold these days. My immune system improved from walking that much.'

Sometimes, he says, the annual health checks required by the law flag up that the weight of one of his employees is swelling. When that happens, the government pays to refer them to a specialist who will see them over six months, and they can provide them with coaching and support to turn their health around. In his company, 100 per cent of the people referred to counselling complete the course and see positive outcomes. But if a company fails and has a fattening workforce, it can be fined. For example, NEC, Japan's biggest manufacturer of electronics, estimated it could face $19 million in fines for the poor health of its workforce, and introduced extensive changes as a result.

Junya said that no individual is forced to do anything as a result of this law. 'You never say "do this". Right? The ideal is that people actually realise their condition. Their health is maybe deteriorating, and they can see that and take control over their health. In this company, we say "measure, understand, realise and change".' He said that his employees can see the data on what everyone else eats and does for exercise because 'it is very hard to continue a routine on your own. If you see everybody else is doing it, you are motivated to take part. You can see the company president' – he gestured towards himself – 'included in that. The president is busy. He's also trying to walk a lot ... Everybody knows that obesity leads to serious illnesses. This is evidence-based. It is also shown by the state and the government. So even if you are healthy, you should watch out for the future, so you can prevent any further potential illnesses. Right now, it might be okay to be obese, but in ten or fifteen years' time, you will suffer. Is that okay with you? I think that's the question.'

I spoke with some of his employees. One 33-year-old man named Yusuke Nagira told me he came to work here straight from university, and he had never done anything to look after his health up to that point. 'I would eat whatever I wanted to eat and didn't exercise at all. That was my lifestyle.' But he noticed from logging his weight that he was getting fatter, and he was conscious of the looming annual health checks. So he made some changes. Before, 'when I was watching TV, I would usually eat junk food or snacks'. He cut them out completely. And 'when I go out to other places, I try not to use trains or drive, but walk'. Knowing he'll be accountable helps him, he said. I heard this again and again from the workers.

I told all the Japanese people I talked to that if you tried this in the US or Britain, people would be outraged and burn down their offices. They invariably looked puzzled, and asked me why.

I said that people would feel like it was not their employer's business what they weighed, and that it was a monstrous intrusion on their privacy. Most of them nodded politely, said nothing, and looked at me like I was slightly crazy. Yusuke said simply: 'Being fat is not good.' I felt like I was communicating across a cultural chasm.

This also left me feeling confused about stigma. The evidence is very clear that once somebody is obese, stigma is a terrible tool to make them change, and actually makes them likely to eat more and exercise less. But I wondered if Japan's experience suggests that stigma has some preventative effect. I felt uncomfortable even asking this question, because I dislike stigma so much.

Whatever you think of its ethics, the Metabo Law does seem to be – along with Japan's other measures – having an impact. The country's obesity rate is currently the lowest in the developed world.

~

It was slowly becoming clear to me that Japanese people put huge cultural barriers between them and overeating. Of course, there are some branches of KFC and McDonald's, and you can eat there three times a day if you want to – but at every stage of life, together, they prevent each other from doing that. Fast food is a treat, not a staple.

As we travelled across the country, Adam and I began to see what you gain if you live in the Japanese style. Every morning around 7 or 8 a.m., in parks across Japan, elderly people gather in groups and exercise together. You can watch people in their eighties and nineties dancing or doing yoga. Japanese people live longer than anyone else on earth. On average, men live to be eighty-one, and women reach eighty-six. Even more importantly, they remain healthy for much longer. The average American and British person is in poor health for between sixteen and nineteen years before they die. In Japan, it's five to six years. They have far fewer heart attacks, and while one in seven British women and one in eight American women get breast cancer, in Japan, it's just one in thirty-eight.

In Kobe, I went to meet members of a football team for men in their eighties and nineties, who compete against other people in an organised league across Japan. A man named Yukio Morimoto, who is eighty-one, told me he now he plays football three times a week. When he started to play again in his sixties – an age at which most Westerners are giving up vigorous exercise – he discovered that 'I felt the same excitement as when I fell in love for the first time. I learned from my teammates. Every day, I was trying to absorb new skills. New tricks.' He told me they are still competitive – if they don't win, he said laughing, they are pissed off. Their teammates in their nineties wear special shorts with turtles and cranes embroidered on them, because in Japanese mythology, turtles are said to live a thousand years, and cranes ten thousand. 'Even though you age,' he said, 'you can maintain your health and your body. Of course, for that, you have to train yourself.' I asked what he eats. 'I have never consciously watched my diet. I just ended up liking what's good for me, and what's good for my body.' His other form of exercise is going dancing with his wife every week. They have been married for fifty-two years.

He leaned towards me and Adam and asked if our elderly relatives play football. We were nonplussed. Adam said the closest we have in Britain is that sometimes men in their fifties get very drunk on a Saturday night, and they will work off their hangovers by kicking a ball around the next day. The Japanese footballers fell into a polite silence.

But to some Japanese people, even these footballers look like whippersnappers. We travelled to Okinawa, an archipelago of islands in the far south of the country, to track down somewhere that sounds almost mythical – the village with the oldest population in the world. By the side of a lush tree-covered mountain, we drove into a village named Ogimi. It has 215 households, and 173 people there are ninety or older. The people who live here have had hard lives – they were mostly poor farmers, and during the war, in the space of just three months, roughly a third of the population was killed during the Battle of Okinawa. Yet by some calculations, nobody in the world lives longer than they do.

In their little concrete community centre, some of the very elderly residents were arriving, looking forward to catching up with each other, playing games and exercising together. The first person we met was Matsu Fukuchi, a 102-year-old woman, who had walked to the centre from her home, slowly but without a stoop, holding on to a cane. Her face was a perfect crumple of wrinkles, and staring out from it, her eyes watched us with curiosity. She wasn't staying for long today, she explained, because she was looking after her 74-year-old son who was recovering after he fell off a roof a few months before. 'I grew up in the mountains,' she told me, and worked as a bamboo farmer for decades, physically harvesting the crop and carrying it down to the market to be sold. She said she took a lot of pleasure in life. 'I get together with my grandchildren and have fun, and dance. I love to dance. I like to watch sports too – basketball, volleyball, sumo. This is the season right now, so I'm watching TV all the time ... Everybody asks me how to live so long. But to me, it's just natural. It just happened naturally. I was always poor. Growing up, I ate potato leaves, and miso soup, and soft-cooked rice. I haven't really paid attention to my health. But I eat vegetables.'

The group started to play games – they had a contest of rock, paper, scissors, which I joined in, and lost. Then some traditional Okinawan music began to play, and Matsu put on a brightly coloured kimono. Then slowly, carefully, joyfully, she stood up, and began to dance. She moved her hips gently in time with the music, and the other women matched her rhythm, waving their arms. She looked towards me and beamed so hard that her eyes almost vanished in her face.

As I watched these women as old as a century moving in time with the music, I felt choked with emotion. Suddenly I realised – *this* is what this whole journey has been about. If you get your health right, if you learn how to eat, if you defeat obesity, if your knees and heart and pancreas are not ruined, then you can have more life, and more health. My grandmother, my friend Hannah, all the people I loved who were diminished or killed too soon by obesity – they should have had all this. It is what I wanted for my godson Adam – a long life, full of health. Matsu was born the year before radio broadcasting began, and on that day, I recorded our conversation on an iPhone.

While she waved her 102-year-old hips in my direction, I thought: This is the potential prize here. More life. More health. More years of joy.

~

One night, shortly before we left Japan, Adam and I did something that, at first glance, sounds insane. We went to a rough part of Tokyo controlled primarily by the Yakuza, the organised crime group, to find a little wooden restaurant named Uoshou. When we stepped in, a tiny woman in her eighties greeted us and ushered us to a small, low table. The clientele for this restaurant, we had been told, are mostly gangsters and prostitutes, and they come here for the speciality of the house – one that many people are too scared to eat. There is a freshwater fish in Japan known as 'fugu', and it is regarded as one of the most delicious delicacies in the whole country – but there's a catch. It's an extraordinarily poisonous pufferfish, with ovaries that are thirteen times more deadly to humans than arsenic. Every year, two or three people die after eating fugu that has not been properly prepared. The chef, Osamu Iimura, told me that it's a terrible death. 'It attacks your neurons,' he said. 'You can't move. Then it attacks your respiratory system,' and you slowly suffocate. 'But until the end, your mind is clear.'

He stressed that as a trained chef, he knew how to cook it, and has a licence granted by the city to do so – but then he chuckled in a disconcerting way. An hour later, the fugu arrived, and Adam and I stared at each other and at the cooked fish. The chef told me to eat the fugu's mouth first – so I looked at its blubbery Mick Jagger lips, took a bite and swallowed hard. It was, indeed, delicious – full of a strange flavour I had never known before. I monitored my breathing. Was I asphyxiating? Adam took his turn next, eating a lump of its white flesh. And on we went, carefully chewing.

As we slowly and delicately ate this killer, it occurred to me: Even this, the most dangerous food in Japan, is safer than the food we eat every day in the West. Junk food, processed food and the obesity they produce kill 112,000 Americans a year at least. Fugu kills a handful of the Japanese. I said to Adam: 'I should feel more anxious eating at McDonald's or when I chow down on a ready-made lasagne than I do here, eating fugu and waiting for signs of death.'

~

When we walked into Tokyo Haneda Airport to board our flight home, Adam looked thoughtful. 'Eating Japanese food for two weeks has made me realise …' He hesitated for a moment. 'It's made me realise how shit the food I've eaten all my life really is.' He said that at home, he frequently has terrible constipation and stomach pains, but within a few days here, these symptoms had gone. 'I don't want to be one of those wankers who says to people "Oh, you're eating *that*? Well, when I was in Japan …" But, God, we need to learn from this.' Suddenly, the sheer artificiality of the obesity crisis seemed clear to me, more than at any other point on this journey. It is created by the way we live. It should be possible, therefore, to un-create it.

But how can we do that? At first glance, the gap between us and the Japanese seemed unbridgeable. But then I thought about something from my own childhood. I told Adam that if I could take him back to the Britain or the United States of (say) 1987, he would be astonished by one thing, more than anything else. People smoked cigarettes *everywhere.* They smoked in restaurants. They smoked on planes. They smoked on game shows. When you went to see the doctor, he would smoke while he examined you. (I'm not kidding: I remember this happening.) There's a photograph of me and my mother, when I am a baby. She's breastfeeding me, smoking, and resting the ashtray on my stomach. (When I found this photo a few years ago and showed it to her, she said: 'You were a fucking difficult baby. I needed that cigarette.')

If you had said to people in 1987 that within a generation, smoking would have almost vanished, we would not have believed you. In 1982, 71 per cent of men and 54 per cent of women were smokers. Today, only 12 per cent of people are smokers, and it's falling further. The British government is about to slowly criminalise the sale of cigarettes. Almost none of Adam's friends smoke them. This is an enormous cultural transformation, in a very short period of time.

I had asked Masaru Watanabe, the Japanese chef, if it was possible for Westerners to become like the Japanese. 'I hope so,' he said. 'I definitely think so.'

As our plane took off, I thought about all the places in the world where I had seen, over the years, the first steps that could be taken to begin this cultural change. I had been in Mexico in 2015 just after they introduced a tax on sugary drinks, pushing up the price of the most unhealthy sodas. In most places where this has been tried, it has reduced purchases of these drinks. We could go much further, taxing processed foods, and using the money to subsidise healthy foods and make them more affordable for everyone.

I went to Amsterdam in 2019, where the mayor launched a major initiative to bring down childhood obesity, by banning unhealthy food in schools, replacing soda and sugary juices with tap water, hugely increasing exercise programmes, and by providing compassionate personal coaches to parents with obese kids to help them find solutions at home. They focused help on the poorest children, who had the biggest problem. In just four years, they cut childhood obesity by 12 per cent across the board, and by 18 per cent for the poorest kids.

In Minneapolis, I visited a team of doctors who could see that the way we eat was making their patients sick. Teaming up with a local charity, they began to 'prescribe' free supplies of healthy food to their patients. Sarah Kempainen, one of the doctors involved in the programme, told me: 'How are people able to stay healthy or prevent disease? It's largely by having access to healthy food … so food *is* medicine.' A study showed that after six months, her patients felt significantly healthier. We could do this on a mass scale.

In Britain, I met with the blood pressure expert Graham MacGregor, who persuaded the food companies to dramatically reduce the amount of salt in their bread – a simple change that nobody noticed when it came to taste. It saves between 6,000 and 9,000 lives a year from strokes in the UK alone. He told me that this approach – of reformulating the recipes of popular foods in our supermarkets – is spreading all over the world, and could be used with many more foods. The best way to achieve it is through governments regulating the food industry.

I interviewed a scientist from Finland named Pekka Puska, who investigated why his country had the highest rate of heart attacks in the world after his own father was killed by one. It turned out to be because they ate a catastrophic diet full of extreme saturated fats and lots of salt. He launched a campaign to transform how people ate – educating the public about the risks, persuading food companies to change their ingredients, and launching a mass programme of volunteers to teach people how to cook differently. As a direct result, Finnish men became 80 per cent less likely to die of heart disease. It increased life expectancy in the North Karelia region, where these changes began, by ten years, and by seven years in the rest of Finland.

As I watched Japan disappear beneath the clouds, I realised that it is not true to say that, in the medium to long term, the only choice we face is between obesity and the new weight-loss drugs. There is a third option. We can become more like Japan, and all these other places. But the Japanese mother who I showed photos of our school lunches to had asked the key question: Is there a movement to do this? Are people fighting for it? This will never be handed down from on high. It will only happen if enough of us demand it.

I turned and looked down the aisle of the plane. Adam was resting his head on a neck pillow, and was already drifting off to sleep. He looked so different from when he had weighed eight stone more, only a few years before. His skin had a healthy glow, and he was breathing easily. I wondered: Are we going to build a culture that makes it as easy as possible for him to stay like this – or one that sabotages him at every turn?

Conclusion: *The Choices Now*
So what do we do, for us, and our kids?

Slowly, as I have worked on this book, my internal conflict has faded a little, and I have begun to have a firmer position on these weight-loss drugs. It is still complex, but it was becoming increasingly clear.

My first conviction is that we need to radically change the kind of food we are given from an early age, so the next generation doesn't become hooked on shitty, satiety-sapping foods and they don't feel the need to drug themselves to escape them. There are risks to the weight-loss drugs; there are no risks to becoming more like the Japanese. Since you've been on this journey with me, I doubt there are many of you who do not believe that now, unless you work for the processed food industry.

But my second conviction is that while we fight for that to happen, in the meantime I still face a choice. I don't live in a better future. I live in the imperfect present, and here, I have to weigh the risks of being obese against the risks posed by these drugs. If I had continued to be as obese as I was at the start of 2023, with 32 per cent body fat, I would be significantly more likely to develop diabetes, knee and hip problems, arthritis, cancer, cognitive problems leading to dementia, high blood pressure leading to a stroke, or – like my grandfather – to die young of a heart attack. It's tempting to ignore the overwhelming scientific evidence for this, but if I do, the only person I'm cheating is myself. These drugs have reversed my obesity, and I can feel how they have improved my health. I walk faster; I don't get breathless; I feel more agile and freer in my whole body. I feel like I have physically healed.

Yet I am also conscious that the drugs bring significant risks of their own. There are the side effects: I still get a little nauseous about once a week, and every few days, I have an unpleasant bout of feeling light-headed and a bit dizzy that lasts a few minutes. It's hard to shake off the feeling this is a sign from my body that something is wrong. The evidence that these drugs increase the low risk you'll get thyroid cancer by 56 per cent is sobering. I am carefully monitoring my muscle mass so it doesn't dip and leave me more frail as I get older: it hasn't fallen yet, but for lots of people on these drugs, it does. It's possible the longer-term warnings – about depression, or suicide, or some as-yet-unidentified danger – will turn out to be true. Since I started taking Ozempic, I have definitely felt more muted in my emotions, though it would be going too far to say I've been depressed. I am assuming that's because I miss the psychological role that overeating used to play in my life, comforting and soothing me, and I'm trying to find other ways to meet those needs, step by step. But I can't know that for sure. Maybe the drug is creating this effect in my brain. I can't dismiss that fear.

I have also become a bit wary of my own judgement, after my friend Lara challenged me about my motives. I am aware that in addition to boosting my health, these drugs bring me more into line with the conventional idea of what it means to be good-looking. I am still not sure if this is skewing my reasoning, and tilting it in favour of the drugs. It might be.

But after thinking about this a lot, I have tentatively concluded that, for me, the benefits outweigh the risks, and for that reason, I'm going to carry on taking these drugs for the foreseeable future. The advice I started to offer other people was: if your BMI is lower than 27, you definitely shouldn't take these drugs. If your BMI is higher than 35, and you don't have a family history of thyroid cancer, and you're not trying to get pregnant, you should probably take these drugs. If your BMI is between 27 and 35, it's more of a finely balanced debate. But I am also conscious that lots of reasonable people will look at the same facts I have looked at, and reach different conclusions on this.

My third conviction is that, whatever you decide for yourself, we should be urgently putting measures in place to prevent some of the problems these drugs will cause for more vulnerable people. I remain really worried about people with eating disorders using these drugs to try to achieve their goal of starving themselves. We can't prevent it entirely, but we can do a lot to limit it. We need to stop these drugs from being prescribed online. To get them, you should have to go, in person, to a doctor who is trained in detecting eating disorders.

So with these three convictions, I thought I had the moral finale for this book. Fight for an environment where we don't face the bleak choice between obesity and drugs; for now, carefully weigh the risks when making a decision for yourself; and fight for measures to protect people with eating disorders.

But then something happened, and it ripped the dilemma of these drugs open for me all over again.

~

As people all over the world started to experience radical weight loss on these drugs, a new question was posed by doctors, parents and teachers.

Should we give them to teenagers too?

Should we give them to kids?

By radically raising the stakes, this dilemma reopened all my doubts. As an adult, I can choose to take a risk with my own health, knowing that the person who will pay the price if I turn out to be wrong is me. But when we make these decisions for a child, we are determining the health of another person. The drugs only work for as long as you take them, so if you drug a child, you're deciding they'll likely be on an expensive medication for the rest of their lives – which could mean seventy or eighty years. If I was assessing this risk not for me but for a ten-year-old, would I feel the same?

I only really understood how hard this choice is when I interviewed Debra Tyler. She's a nurse in Connecticut, and her daughter – who I'll call Anna – started to gain a lot of weight when she was very young. 'She's always been a big eater,' she told me. 'She just never feels full.' Anna was always running around and exercising – she would often go swimming and ride horses – but because of her weight, she struggled to keep up with the other kids. Debra knew where this could lead, because she had seen it in other family members. Her husband had been very overweight and had a heart attack when he was forty-five, and two of his brothers had died of cardiac problems. But she didn't expect what happened next.

When Anna was five years old, a doctor checked her cholesterol and found that her lipids were very high. She was immediately referred to an endocrine specialist, who was alarmed and advised Debra to urgently change Anna's diet. Debra really worked at it, but found 'it's hard with a kid, because they don't understand … It was a daily struggle.' She tried encouraging her daughter to eat all sorts of healthier foods and try out different forms of exercise, like basketball. 'It was a lot of trying to figure out how to help her – and really, none of it worked, to be honest. It was always a struggle. And then you feel guilty. Like – oh my gosh, what have we done?'

As Anna's weight began to approach two hundred pounds in her early teens, the signs of her underlying health got even worse. She was referred to a programme designed to help divert kids away from developing diabetes, and the initial tests found that Anna's liver was also in trouble. 'She went from a fatty liver of 7 per cent to 21 per cent, and the doctor said she [was] almost [certainly] going to need a liver specialist, so we needed to do something.' Her cholesterol was also dangerously high.

When Debra heard about Ozempic, all her instincts were against it. 'The last thing I wanted to do was put my kid on medicine,' she said. She was worried that it might make Anna feel ashamed of her body. 'I didn't want to create an eating disorder. I didn't want her to be a closet eater, or an anorexic.' But she had tried the obvious solutions of diet and exercise many times. So Anna began to be injected once a week with the drug. For the first few days, she had mild nausea, then it went away. 'Pretty quickly, we noticed that her appetite had slowed down,'

Debra said. Anna became dramatically less obese, and her liver functioning rapidly returned to a healthy level. Debra was happy to see her daughter getting better – but still uneasy.

Then, one day, Debra went to the pharmacy to collect the next dose of Ozempic, and the pharmacist told her that because her work health insurance had changed, Anna was no longer eligible for the drug. She had to come off it, and within a few weeks, her appetite was back to its old levels. Debra knew what would likely come next: a deteriorating liver. So she and her husband made a painful decision. They decided to buy Wegovy (the same drug as Ozempic, but branded for obesity) out of their own pockets, at more than $800 a month. We are, she said, 'trying to prevent her becoming diabetic. That's the main reason – just for her health.'

But she told me that she's still unsure about this decision. Nobody knows the long-term effects of these drugs on kids. It's a literal experiment. She's switched the whole family to a vegan diet, and they're all losing some weight now. When I asked her about the need to tackle the wider causes of obesity in our society, she was sympathetic, but said: 'Good luck fighting the food industry, because you're not going to win. There's not going to be a change in food, for political and money reasons.'

The conflict Debra is experiencing is one that many parents are facing. Her dilemma was extreme, because her daughter's obesity – and the risk to her health – was so acute and she was so young. But childhood obesity has been exploding throughout my lifetime, even more than among adults. If you're over forty and you go to any playground in the US or Britain, you'll notice the kids look really different compared to how they did when you were at school. In a single decade, the number of obese kids in Britain shot up by 70 per cent. In the US, the rate of increase in childhood obesity doubled during the pandemic years. This has happened in part because fast-food companies have consciously targeted our children. Today, 67 per cent of the food calories consumed by kids in the US come from ultra-processed foods.

Giles Yeo, the obesity expert at Cambridge University, told me: 'When you have obesity as a child, it's very difficult to become un-obese … The likelihood is therefore you end up with obesity for life, or for a long part of life.' The effects on children's health of obesity have been investigated by scientists, and they are often horrifying. A summary of the evidence was published in *Pediatrics*, the journal of the American Academy of Pediatrics, in 2023. It explained: 'Obesity puts children and adolescents at risk for serious short- and long-term adverse health outcomes later in life, including cardiovascular disease; dyslipidemia; insulin resistance; T2DM [type 2 diabetes]; and nonalcoholic fatty liver disease.' These are some of the biggest killers in our society.

So it's not hard to see why some scientists said we should experiment with giving weight-loss drugs to teens. They argue that if you can reverse obesity early, you will likely improve that kid's health across their whole lifespan. The largest clinical trial on young people took 134 adolescents aged between twelve and seventeen who had become obese and gave them the drugs. Their weight loss was dramatic. After sixty-eight weeks, nearly half of them had fallen below the threshold for obesity, and a quarter got all the way to the healthy weight for their age. After a year on these drugs, 62 per cent of the obese kids lost at least 10 per cent of their body weight – a startling outcome when you consider they were still growing. The co-author of the first study, Aaron Kelly – who is co-director of the Center for Pediatric Obesity Medicine at the University of Minnesota – told an interviewer that these results are 'historically unprecedented with treatments other than bariatric surgery'.

The upside is clear. Just as Debra watched the warning signs that were flashing around her daughter Anna's health begin to fade away, those kids are also much less likely to develop diabetes, cardiovascular disease and liver problems. However, the clinical trials found that the side effects were real too. Sixty-two per cent of the kids in that larger trial experienced nausea or upset stomachs. They lasted, on average, for two or three days, then mostly went away – though more long-lasting nausea or upset stomachs happened in 11 per cent of the kids.

This evidence encouraged a wave of optimism about giving these drugs to teens. But some other doctors – equally reputable and sincere – then tried to pull the emergency brake on rolling them out across the world's playgrounds. For example, Dan Cooper, a professor of paediatrics at the University of California, Irvine, and his colleagues wrote a paper warning that 'children are not miniature adults'. Giving these drugs to people who are still developing poses a whole new set of risks – ones that wouldn't have emerged in the adult trials, and may be very serious. To develop properly, children need a lot of calories, but these weight-loss drugs can cause 'unbalanced and inappropriate reductions in caloric (energy) intake'. If a kid's incoming calories suddenly contract to below a healthy level, it could stunt their growth – and it could cause other health problems. Children use calories for bone mineralisation, which is a key part of the process of forming healthy bones. If this doesn't happen properly because the calories came down too hard, they are at greater risk of osteoporosis later in life.

In addition, kids with eating disorders could get hold of these drugs and really harm themselves. They said the danger of this is even greater now, because social media has supercharged the trend for kids feeling bad about their bodies, creating 'a perfect storm for potential abuse'. Telling a child there's something wrong with their body that requires lifelong drugging is a serious step, with unpredictable consequences for their sense of who they are.

There's an obvious further danger, one this group of scientists didn't raise. We don't currently know the risk to adults of taking these drugs to treat obesity for ten or twenty years – so we have absolutely no idea about the risk of what will happen to children who will be potentially taking it for eighty years.

Dan and his colleagues argued that rather than giving out drugs, we should stop 'medicalizing pediatric conditions, many of which emerge from environmental and societal rather than biological mechanisms', and instead address 'the environmental and lifestyle issues that have contributed immeasurably to the childhood obesity epidemic'.

These concerns are going to become even more acute, as some scientists make the case for rolling out the drugs to younger and younger children.

As I write this, Novo Nordisk is carrying out a clinical trial on giving them to children as young as six.

~

I tried to imagine having an obese child and deciding whether to drug them or not. But I kept being overwhelmed by an emotion that I had kept at bay for most of the writing of this book – a biting anger.

Why is this the choice we are faced with: leave your kids with a dangerous physical condition that could trash their health, or give them a potentially dangerous drug for ever? How did we come to this? It didn't happen by accident. We allowed the food industry, unregulated, to wreck our kids' health. There's a huge amount of evidence for this, but I'll pluck, at random, one piece of it. An internal memo was released in 1998 from a company that makes a lot of the biscuits you've probably eaten. They wrote that they had spoken with the most famous names in the fast-food industry, to figure out the best way to market to kids. They concluded: 'It is important to note that since taste preferences are determined early, a great deal of effort focuses [on those] even younger than teen.' To achieve this, these companies 'focus on children's movies and TV characters', and donate materials with their logos to schools as well as fast food for their school lunch programmes – all to get kids craving their products as early and as often as possible.

The memo, like the industry, is built around getting kids to hoover up shitty food that will make them sick, so these companies can make more money. They spend more than a billion dollars a year in the US alone marketing to kids. This was done to me, throughout my childhood, and it made me consume this crap and learn to love it. This should never have happened. We should, in democratic societies, have regulated the companies, to stop it happening. We can start now. Our kids deserve better than to have their tastes and their health hijacked for profit.

~

So what will happen now? After everything I've learned, I think there are essentially five possible scenarios for how these drugs will play out. I'll start with the most pessimistic, and work my way up to optimism – then I'll tell you which I think is most likely.

The first scenario is that this is fen-phen Mark 2. Perhaps there is a disastrous effect of these drugs that we have only glimpsed so far. It could be connected to the safety signals about thyroid cancer and suicidal thoughts that have already been raised in the European Union, or perhaps it's something we haven't spotted yet. This obscure or unknown effect would have to be very severe to outweigh the effects of obesity, but we have been here with a diet drug before, only thirty years ago, so only a fool would dismiss this possibility.

The second scenario is that these drugs are like chemical antidepressants. They produce a big effect at first, but for most people, the effect fades away over time. Some people taking chemical antidepressants experience a long-lasting boost (and if you're one of those people, my advice is to carry on taking them) – but sadly, the best long-term trial of the drugs found that most people slowly become depressed again over time. That's what happened to me when I took Paxil, a popular SSRI antidepressant. It's possible that, similarly, the decline in weight caused by these drugs will fade over five or ten years, so a decade from now, I'll be back to the weight I would have been if Ozempic had never been invented.

The third scenario is that they are like the statins we are prescribed for heart problems. These heart-protecting drugs block a substance that your body needs to produce cholesterol, so when you take them, your cholesterol levels fall dramatically. Statins do not deal with the underlying reasons why people have heart attacks – stress, poor diet, lack of exercise – but nonetheless, by dealing with one of the intermediate biological mechanisms, they prevent a huge number of heart attacks, and have almost certainly saved the life of somebody you love. The new weight-loss drugs could come to be seen like this. But there's a catch to this comparison.

Statins are really cheap to manufacture, and as a result, they are the most prescribed drug in many rich countries. At the moment, we couldn't roll out the new weight-loss drugs like that even if we wanted to, because they are enormously expensive. If we were going to give them to every person who's eligible (70 per cent of the population in the US), they would risk bankrupting state-run or private health insurance programmes. Walter Willett, the Harvard professor I interviewed earlier, has warned that giving these drugs to everyone who qualifies for them could add 50 per cent to existing healthcare budgets. This is not because of the inherent cost of these drugs – they can be manufactured for as little as $40 a month. It's because the copyright on the drugs is owned by Novo Nordisk and Eli Lilly, who argue that because they put in the risky investment to develop them, they should rake in the rewards. That's why they are charging up to $1,200 a month in the US.

So there's a risk that these drugs are a real lifesaver, but they are restricted to a small elite, while the rest of the population will continue to become increasingly obese and die sooner than they had to. The Real Housewives of New Jersey will get to be thin, while the real schoolkids of New Jersey will develop diabetes at twelve.

The fourth scenario is both that these drugs are like statins *and* that over time they will be provided to anyone who needs them. Different countries could expand access in different ways. Britain has a National Health Service funded through general taxes, so perhaps they will buy and distribute them in bulk for a lower price, knowing it will save a fortune in health costs further down the road. In the United States, there's a few ways this could play out. Perhaps competition between different weight-loss drugs will drive down prices. Maybe the companies will figure that they can make more money if they sell these drugs for less at a very large scale. It's also possible these drugs will spur further efforts to regulate the pharmaceutical companies and compel them to charge less.

In any event, by 2032, the copyright on many of these drugs will have expired, which means anyone will be able to manufacture cheap generic versions for $40 a month or so. If these drugs become widely, cheaply and safely available, it could be an extraordinary turning point. We might look back decades from now and say: because of a lousy food system, we fell into an obesity crisis, but then a drug pulled many of us out of the ditch and reversed a great deal of the harm.

Then there's a fifth scenario – the most optimistic. It's that many of us start to take these drugs, and experience significant weight loss, and see our health improve – and it wakes us up to ask: how did we get into this situation in the first place? How did we end up with a food system so dysfunctional that we need to engage in a programme of mass drugging to protect us from it? Do we want our kids to have to drug themselves in this way? The people of Japan don't need these drugs, so why do we? Who stole our satiety, and how do we stop them stealing it from the next generation, so they don't have to take this drastic step as well? The extraordinary need for these drugs could trigger a moment of shock and self-understanding, and spur the creation of a movement to deal with the underlying factors that caused this crisis in the first place.

After everything I've learned from researching this book, it's daunting to know that we are still not sure which of these scenarios will turn out to be the case. These drugs could be a killer, or they could be the beginning of the end of the obesity crisis. If you put a gun to my head and forced me to say which scenario I think is most likely to come to pass, I would name the third, or fourth. But I'm going to fight for number five. I hope you'll join me.

~

There's only one photo of my friend Hannah on the internet. It was taken a few years before she died of a heart attack in her mid-forties, after a lifetime of being obese. It's the profile picture from her Twitter feed. She's staring into the camera with that facial expression I saw so often, but even now, I struggle to describe it. She is almost laughing, but not quite. There's a trace of fear around her eyes, but also a determination in her mouth that she is going kill that fear with a brilliant quip. The stakes in dealing with the obesity crisis are very high – millions of people will live or die, depending on whether we get this right. She's the one I can't forget. If we'd got this right a generation ago, I believe she would be here now.

But if she was, I know she'd say: 'Stakes? It's steaks I want, you moaning twat. Now open Uber Eats, switch on *Judge Judy*, and stop all this whining.'

I didn't forget you, Hannah.

I miss you.

And I won't forget what killed you.

WHAT YOU CAN DO TO IMPROVE THE FOOD SYSTEM

There are several groups that are fighting to improve the food system – I urge you to support them! Here's a few:

IN THE US

Healthy Schools Campaign: https://healthyschoolscampaign.org/issues/school-food/
School Food Matters: https://www.schoolfoodmatters.org/
The Food Research and Action Centre: https://frac.org/healthy-school-meals-for-all
Food and Water Watch: https://www.foodandwaterwatch.org/who-we-are/
Black Urban Growers: www.blackurbangrowers.com

IN THE UK

Food Foundation: https://foodfoundation.org.uk/

IN AUSTRALIA

Food for Health Alliance: https://www.foodforhealthalliance.org.au/

I CAN KEEP YOU POSTED

If you'd like to receive occasional email updates from me with information about developments on the fight to improve the food system, or the evolving science around these new weight-loss drugs, please go to www.magicpillbook.com/updates.

FURTHER READING

There are several books I'd recommend if you want to learn more about some of the themes in this book. If you want to understand more about what processed food is doing to us, I recommend *Ultra-Processed People* by Chris van Tulleken, *Swallow This* by Joanna Blythman, *Food for Life* by Tim Spector, *Ravenous* by Henry Dimbleby and *In Defence of Food* by Michael Pollan. To discover more about trauma and how it can affect our bodies, I recommend *In the Body of the World* by V (formerly known as Eve Ensler), *On Our Best Behaviour* by Elise Loehnen and *Hunger* by Roxane Gay. To hear about the science of how obesity affects our bodies, *Conquering Fat Logic* by the German nutritionist Nadja Hermann is very good. To see more about how we can build a sustainable movement to end stigma, I recommend *The Forbidden Body* and *What Have You Got to Lose?* by Shelley Bovey. To learn how to cook and be healthier, any book by Rangan Chatterjee is great: I'd recommend starting with *Feel Good.*

The food writer Bee Wilson is very insightful – her book *First Bite*, about how children develop their tastes, is particularly excellent, and I'd recommend it to all parents. If you're curious about Japanese food, *Sushi and Beyond* by Michael Booth is a charming travel book on this subject.

And throughout this book, I have drawn on areas of science I learned about for two of my previous books: *Chasing the Scream*, which is about why we become addicted and what we can do about it, and *Lost Connections*, which is about the reasons why depression and anxiety have risen and how we can reverse them.

ACKNOWLEDGEMENTS

I'm really grateful to all the people who supported me while I was writing this book and made it possible. My editors Kevin Doughten and Alexis Kirschbaum were brilliant, and so were my agents, Natasha Fairweather and Richard Pine. Sarah Punshon, Jake Hess and Sean Lavery were my fact-checkers, and conversations with them produced lots of the insights that you've read here: I am very much in their debt. My wonderful friends Elizabeth Davidson and Decca Aitkenhead were particularly helpful in discussing these subjects with me at great length.

Katie Aitken-Quack and Patricia Clark, the lawyers for my publishers, did an excellent job, as did my copyeditor, Katherine Fry, and my wonderful production manager, Lauren Whybrow.

In Japan, my fixer was Chie Matsumoto; in Iceland, I was helped by Halldór Árnason and his family; in Denmark, Jonas Ejlersen carried out some translation for me; and in the Netherlands, Rosanne Kropmann did the same. I am thankful to all of them.

I am really thankful to all the scientists and experts who shared their expertise with me. I am also hugely indebted to Naomi Klein, V (formerly known as Eve Ensler), Ben Hari, Jerome Johnson, Rosie Tasker, Jemima Goldsmith, Elisa Hari, Aaron Hari, Erin Hari, Josh Wood, Steph Sharkey, Isaac Wood, Deborah Friedell, Stephen Grosz, Rosie Tasker, Amy

Li, Jessica Luxembourg, Rob Blackhurst, Andrew Sullivan, Patrick Strudwick, Ronan McCrea, Tristan Kendrick, Laurence Laluyaux, Stephen Edwards, Katharina Volckmer, Barbara Bateman and Hermione Lawton.

My Patreon supporters, through their generosity, make it possible for me to take the time to do the deep research my books require. I want to particularly thank Pam Roy, Erik de Bruijn, Rachel Bomgaars, Lynn McFarland, Nicole Collins and Stephen Duke. If you'd like to join them, and receive regular updates about what I'm researching and working on next, please go to https://www.patreon.com/johannhari.

My description of my time in the Mayr Clinic is partially taken from an article I wrote about it for the *Independent* in 2007. Thank you to the newspaper for giving permission for me to use this material.

All errors in this book are mine alone. If you spot any, please email me at chasingthescream@gmail.com and I'll correct them in future editions and thank you on the website. All corrections will be posted at www.magicpillbook.com/corrections.

NOTES

Please note these are partial endnotes. I have only included the most important studies here, because (oh the irony) I didn't want this book to be too fat.

There are more than 30,000 words of additional notes on the book's website, explaining a lot more of the context to the science I have discussed here, and many other things I think it will help you to know. Please go to www.magicpillbook.com/endnotes.

Also, on that part of the website, you can hear the audio for the conversations you've read about in this book. They are embedded throughout the Notes section.

INTRODUCTION: THE HOLY GRAIL

p. 2 **One afternoon just before Christmas in 2009:** I wrote about this experience in one of my previous books: J. Hari, *Lost Connections: Uncovering the Real Causes of Depression – And the Unexpected Solutions* (Bloomsbury, 2018), p. 91.

p. 3 **Some financial analysts believe that the market for them:** https://www.cnbc.com/2023/04/28/obesity-drugs-to-be-worth-200-billion-in-next-10-years-barclays-says.html, as accessed 18 June 2023; https://companiesmarketcap.com/mcdonald/marketcap/#:~:text=As%20of%20September%202023%20McDonald,cap%20according%20to%20our%20data, as accessed 28 September 2023.

p. 4 **The lowest credible calculation for the US is that it ends 112,000 lives a year:** K. M. Flegal, B. I. Graubard, D. F. Williamson and M. H. Gail, 'Excess Deaths Associated With Underweight, Overweight, and Obesity', *JAMA* (2005), 293(15), pp. 1, 861–7, doi:10.1001/jama.293.15.1861.

p. 4 **At the upper end, Jerold Mande:** This number comes from the 2016 version of the Global Burden of Disease study, as cited by the Center for Science in the Public Interest, 'Why Good Nutrition is Important', undated, https://www.cspinet.org/eating-healthy/why-good-nutrition-important, as accessed 18 October 2022. See also https://harvardpublichealth.org/nutrition/processed-foods-make-us-sick-its-time-for-government-action/#:~:text=Harvard%20professor%20Jerold%20Mande%20argues,and%20USDA%20to%20step%20in.&text=Federal%20food%20law%20is%20clear,food%5D%20injurious%20to%20health.%E2%80%9D, as accessed 10 October 2023.

p. 4 **even the most optimistic studies find that only approximately 20 per cent of us succeed:** This is a rough estimate made by Brown University Medical School researchers based on past studies on dieting and weight loss. See R. R. Wing and S. Phelan, 'Long-term weight loss maintenance', *American Journal of Clinical Nutrition* (2005), 82, suppl. 1, pp. 222S–225S, https://pubmed.ncbi.nlm.nih.gov/16002825/. This is discussed further in Chapter 6.

p. 5 **doubles your risk of dying when you are older:** https://pubmed.ncbi.nlm.nih.gov/16926275/. I first learned about this in the *Oxford Handbook of the Social Science of Obesity* (OUP, 2011), p. 24.

p. 7 **I need to tell you about Hannah:** I have changed Hannah's name and a few minor identifying details here, to respect her and her family's privacy. Because I am describing her from memory, I showed everything I wrote about her to another of her closest friends, Bronwen Carr. She confirmed that this matched her recollections. I also discussed this section with lots of other people who knew Hannah, who agreed that this is, to the best of our knowledge, an accurate picture of her.

p. 7 **I sat down to watch a play called *Atlantica*:** My description of *Atlantica* here is entirely from memory. I tried really hard to locate a text of the play but it seemed to have vanished. Since I'm recalling it from a distance of nearly twenty-five years, I'm sure I'm getting some details wrong, and the dialogue will not be exactly as it appeared in the script. I tracked down everyone I knew who had seen it and asked if this description matched their recollections. They said that broadly it did, though recollections differed a bit from person to person, as you'd expect after all this time. Some of them said that I am wrong to remember that only Hannah and I thought it was absurd, and in fact, a lot of the audience felt the same way. But by contrast, one of the cast members said that it was a more serious play than I remembered, and that lots of people took it seriously.

It's possible we are all remembering it accurately. There were three performances of the play at the festival, and it looks like people at each reacted differently. One critic writing at the time noted that audiences reacted in contrasting ways, writing: 'So that, for instance, *Atlantica*, a new save-the-whale play from Cambridge which blended B-movie and SF elements with an undertow of seriousness reminiscent of the TV series *Edge Of Darkness*, could play to three audiences giving radically different responses from silent seriousness to howls of campy laughter, and accept that each response was both legitimate and respectful on its own terms.' See https://www.cix.co.uk/~shutters/reviews/01091.htm as accessed 20th February 2024.

p. 9 **Socrates whale, slugging hemlock rather than face:** When I reflected on this memory, I had a recollection that in the festival's newsletter, Noises Off, somebody published some sketches of suicidal whales based on famous people. I am not sure if Hannah told the person who drew these sketches this joke, and it was based on what she said; or if Hannah heard this joke from the person who drew them, and she then told it to me. If anyone knows the name of the person who drew them, please let me know, and I'll credit him or her in future editions of the book!

CHAPTER 1 FINDING THE TREASURE CHEST

p. 27 **Svetlana Mojsov worked with a group to put GLP-1 into a rat's pancreas:** S. Mojsov, G. C. Weir and J. F. Habener, 'Insulinotropin: glucagon-like peptide I (7–37) co-encoded in the glucagon gene is a potent stimulator of insulin release in the perfused rat pancreas', *Journal of Clinical Investigation* (1987), 79(2), pp. 616–19, doi:10.1172/JCI112855. See also this fascinating piece for a fuller story of Svetlana Mojsov's involvement in GLP-1 work: https://www.science.org/content/article/her-work-paved-way-blockbuster-obesity-drugs-now-she-s-fighting-recognition#:~:text=1987%3A%20Mojsov%20and%20Habener%2C%20with,listed%20as%20the%20sole%20inventor, as accessed 6 November 2023.

p. 28 **a team in Copenhagen put GLP-1 into a pig's pancreas:** C. Orskov, J. J. Holst and O. V. Nielsen, 'Effect of truncated glucagon-like peptide-1 [proglucagon-(78–107) amide] on endocrine secretion from pig pancreas, antrum, and nonantral stomach', *Endocrinology* (1988), 123, pp. 2,009–13; see also on severe obesity hypoventilation, https://err.ersjournals.com/content/28/151/180097#:~:text=Obesity%20hypoventilation%20syndrome%20(OHS)%20is,that%20may%20cause%20alveolar%20hypoventilation, as accessed 29 October 2023.

p. 29 **He injected GLP-1 into rats, and found that:** https://www.nature.com/articles/379069a0.

p. 30 **a biochemist in the Bronx named John Eng noticed something weird:** J. Eng, 'Exendin peptides', *Mount Sinai Journal of Medicine* (1992), 59, pp. 147–9. See also https://www.diabetesincontrol.com/dr-john-engs-research-found-that-the-saliva-of-the-gila-monster-contains-a-hormone-that-treats-diabetes-better-than-any-other-medicine/, as accessed 28 October 2023.

p. 32 **the official results of their major trial giving semaglutide to obese people:** J. P. H. Wilding et al., 'Once-Weekly Semaglutide in Adults with Overweight or Obesity', *New England Journal of Medicine* (2021), 384(11), pp. 989–1,002, doi:10.1056/NEJMoa2032183.

p. 33 **after they quit, most people regain two-thirds of the weight they lost within a year:** https://dom-pubs.onlinelibrary.wiley.com/doi/10.1111/dom.14725.

p. 34 **lost, on average, 21 per cent of their body weight in the clinical trials:** A. M. Jastreboff et al., 'Tirzepatide Once Weekly for the Treatment of Obesity', *New England Journal of Medicine* (2022), 387(3), pp. 205–16, doi:10.1056/NEJMoa2206038, https://www.nejm.org/doi/full/10.1056/NEJMoa2107519. The 20.9 per cent figure is only for the highest dose; weight loss was lower at lower doses.

p. 35 **Early studies suggest it produces 24.2 per cent weight loss:** A. M. Jastreboff et al., 'Triple-Hormone-Receptor Agonist Retatrutide for Obesity – A Phase 2 Trial', *New England Journal of Medicine* (2023), 389(6), pp. 514–26, doi:10.1056/NEJMoa2301972. See also https://www.newscientist.com/article/mg25934470-900-beyond-wegovy-could-the-next-wave-of-weight-loss-drugs-end-obesity/, as accessed 13 August 2023; https://www.reuters.com/business/healthcare-pharmaceuticals/lilly-experimental-triple-g-obesity-drug-leads-242-weight-loss-trial-nejm-2023-06-26/, as accessed 8 October 2023.

p. 35 **two major studies were published that revealed semaglutide pills:** The two main studies: https://www.nejm.org/doi/full/10.1056/NEJMoa2301972; https://www.thelancet.com/journals/lancet/article/PIIS0140-6736(23)01053-X/fulltext.

p. 38 **For many people, when they take these drugs, their resting heart rate increases:** J. Seufert et al., 'Increase in pulse rate with semaglutide did not result in increased adverse cardiac events in subjects with type 2 diabetes in the SUSTAIN 6 cardiovascular outcomes trial', *European Heart Journal* (August 2018), 39, suppl. 1, ehy565.P2857, https://doi.org/10.1093/eurheartj/ehy565.P2857.

p. 39 **For between 5 and 10 per cent of people who take these drugs:** W. T. Garvey et al., 'Two-year effects of semaglutide in adults with overweight or obesity: the STEP 5 trial', *Nature Medicine* (2022), 28, pp. 2,083–91, https://doi.org/10.1038/s41591-022-02026-4. It's not absolutely certain that it's the side effects that are the sole cause of patients not continuing with the drug. STEP 5, for example, had a 92.8 per cent completion rate, but that's averaged across the placebo and semaglutide groups. And in some of the adolescent studies it's almost the exact same drop-out rate for placebo as for the real drug, so more is at work here than side effects.

CHAPTER 2 CHEESECAKE PARK

p. 43 **this began to change in the late 1970s:** See 'The Surgeon General's Vision for a Healthy and Fit Nation' (2010), https://www.ncbi.nlm.nih.gov/books/NBK44656/, as accessed 6 November 2023, for a good summary of studies on this.

p. 43 **Obesity had likely been rising very slowly since the turn of the twentieth century:** J. Komlos and M. Brabec, 'The evolution of BMI values of

US adults: 1882–1986', Center for Economic Policy Research (blog), 31 August 2010, https://cepr.org/voxeu/columns/evolution-bmi-values-us-adults-1882-1986, as accessed 28 September 2023. This study found that BMI began to increase at this time, which is why I say it was 'likely' that obesity rose at this time. BMI and obesity are not synonymous, but they are often closely matched – see the explanation from Walter Willett in Chapter 11.

p. 43 **Between the year I was born and the year I turned twenty-one:** R. Casas, L. Brown and J. Gomez-Ambrosi, 'The Origins of the Obesity Epidemic in the USA – Lessons for Today', *Nutrients* (2022), 14(20), p. 4,253, https://www.ncbi.nlm.nih.gov/pmc/articles/PMC9611578/.

p. 43 **The rate of severe obesity took a particularly disturbing turn:** https://www.cdc.gov/obesity/data/adult.html, as accessed 23 November 2023.

p. 43 **The average American adult weighs twenty-three pounds more than in 1960:** M. Moss, *Sugar Salt Fat* (W. H. Allen, 2014), p. 238; see also S. Gill, 'Is there an average weight for men?', *Medical News Today* (11 October 2014), https://www.medicalnewstoday.com/articles/320917#average-weight-of-men-in-the-us, as accessed 28 October 2023.

p. 43 **more than 70 per cent of all Americans are either overweight or obese:** National Institutes of Health, 'Overweight and Obesity Statistics', September 2021, https://www.niddk.nih.gov/health-information/health-statistics/overweight-obesity, as accessed 26 June 2023.

p. 43 **England has followed a similar trend:** C. Baker, 'Obesity statistics', House of Commons Library, Research Briefing, 12 January 2023, https://researchbriefings.files.parliament.uk/documents/SN03336/SN03336.pdf. See also Tim Spector, *The Diet Myth: The Real Science Behind What We Eat* (Weidenfeld & Nicolson, 2016), p. 12.

p. 43 **the World Health Organization says that obesity has nearly tripled globally:** World Health Organization, 'Obesity and overweight', 9 June 2021, https://www.who.int/news-room/fact-sheets/detail/obesity-and-overweight, as accessed 28 September 2023.

p. 55 **With his colleagues, he designed an experiment to test this:** P. M. Johnson and P. J. Kenny, 'Dopamine D2 receptors in addiction-like reward dysfunction and compulsive eating in obese rats', *Nature Neuroscience* (2010), 13(5), pp. 635–41, https://pubmed.ncbi.nlm.nih.gov/20348917/.

p. 59 **But if you feed them Fruit Loops:** A. Sclafani and D. Springer, 'Dietary obesity in adult rats: Similarities to hypothalamic and human obesity syndromes', *Physiology & Behavior* (1976), 17(3), pp. 461–71, https://www.sciencedirect.com/science/article/abs/pii/0031938476901098. I first learned of Sclafani's experiments in Kessler, *The End of Overeating*, p. 15. See also M. Tordoff, 'Obesity by choice: the powerful influence of nutrient availability on nutrient intake', *American Journal of Physiology-Regulatory, Integrative and Comparatory Physiology*

(2002), 282(5), R1536–R1539, https://pubmed.ncbi.nlm.nih.gov/11959698/, as cited in K. Brownell and K. B. Horgen, *Food Fight* (McGraw Hill, 2003), p. 25.

p. 59 **Barry Levin, a professor at the New Jersey Medical School, bred a strain of rats:** B. E. Levin and A. A. Dunn-Meynell, 'Defense of body weight depends on dietary composition and palatability in rats with diet-induced obesity', *American Journal of Physiology-Regulatory, Integrative and Comparatory Physiology* (2002), 282(1), R46–R54, doi:10.1152/ajpregu.2002.282.1.R46.

CHAPTER 3 THE DEATH AND REBIRTH OF SATIETY

p. 62 **The first glimmer of an answer was discovered in 1995:** S. H. Holt, J. C. Miller, P. Petocz and E. Farmakalidis, 'A satiety index of common foods', *European Journal of Clinical Nutrution* (1995), 49(9), pp. 675–90. I first learned of this study in H. Pontzer, *Burn: The Misunderstood Science of Metabolism* (Penguin, 2021), p. 226.

p. 64 **Chewing, Tim said, is a necessary brake on overeating:** M. Borvornparadorn et al., 'Increased chewing reduces energy intake, but not postprandial glucose and insulin, in healthy weight and overweight young adults', *Nutrition & Dietetics* (2019), 76(1), pp. 89–94, doi:10.1111/1747-0080.12433; Dieuwerke P. Bolhuis and Ciarán G. Forde, 'Application of food texture to moderate oral processing behaviors and energy intake', *Trends in Food Science & Technology* (2020), 106, pp. 445–6, ISSN 0924–2244, https://doi.org/10.1016/j.tifs.2020.10.021. These findings have been used as a weight loss technique, with some success: https://www.researchgate.net/profile/Rebekka-Schnepper/publication/330043007_A_Combined_Mindfulness%27Prolonged_Chewing_Intervention_Reduces_Body_Weight_Food_Craving_and_Emotional_Eating/links/5c2df660a6fdccd6b58f6c99/A-Combined-MindfulnessProlonged-Chewing-Intervention-Reduces-Body-Weight-Food-Craving-and-Emotional-Eating.pdf, as accessed 10 November 2023.

p. 66 **To figure out if this was true, David designed a small but clever experiment:** Stephen J. Simpson, Rachel Batley and David Raubenheimer, 'Geometric analysis of macronutrient intake in humans: the power of protein?', *Appetite* (2003), 41(2), pp. 123–40, ISSN 0195-6663, https://doi.org/10.1016/S0195-6663(03)00049-7. See also C. Wilson, 'What really makes junk food bad for us? Here's what the science says', *New Scientist*, 9 June 2021, https://www.newscientist.com/article/mg25033380-700-what-really-makes-junk-food-bad-for-us-heres-what-the-science-says/, as accessed 1 July 2023; D. Raubenheimer and S. Simpson, 'You have five appetites, not one, and they are the key to your health', *New Scientist*,

20 May 2020, https://www.newscientist.com/article/mg24632831-400-you-have-five-appetites-not-one-and-they-are-the-key-to-your-health/, as accessed 14 August 2023.

p. 66 **the people eating the processed food had to consume 35 per cent more calories:** Simpson, Batley and Raubenheimer, 'Geometric analysis of macronutrient intake in humans'. See also Raubenheimer and Simpson, 'You have five appetites, not one'.

p. 67 **chemicals that may be actively triggering us to be more hungry:** S. E. Swithers, 'Artificial sweeteners produce the counterintuitive effect of inducing metabolic derangements', *Trends in Endocrinology and Metabolism* (2013), 24(9), pp. 431–41, doi:10.1016/j.tem.2013.05.005; L. B. Sorenson et al., 'Sucrose compared with artificial sweeteners: a clinical intervention study of effects on energy intake, appetite, and energy expenditure after 10 wk of supplementation in overweight subjects', *American Journal of Clinical Nutrition* (2014), 100(1), pp. 36–45, https://pubmed.ncbi.nlm.nih.gov/24787495/.

p. 67 **for every extra soft drink a child consumes a day:** D. S. Ludwig, K. E. Peterson and S. L. Gortmaker, 'Relation between consumption of sugar-sweetened drinks and childhood obesity: a prospective, observational analysis', *Lancet* (2001), 357(9255), pp. 505–8, doi:10.1016/S0140-6736(00)04041-1. I first learned about this study in Brownell and Horgen, *Food Fight*, p. 169.

p. 67 **the rats given artificial sweeteners gained *more* weight:** S. E. Swithers and T. L. Davidson, 'A role for sweet taste: calorie predictive relations in energy regulation by rats', *Behavioral Neuroscience* (2008), 122(1), pp. 161–73, doi:10.1037/0735-7044.122.1.161. I first learned about this in Joanna Blythman, *Swallow This: Serving Up the Food Industry's Darkest Secrets* (HarperCollins, 2015), p. 111.

p. 68 **But as Tim watched his glucose levels, he was startled:** Tim Spector, *Spoon Fed: Why Almost Everything We've Been Told About Food is Wrong* (Vintage, 2022), p. 67.

p. 68 **a team of Israeli scientists split 120 people:** J. Suez et al., 'Personalized microbiome-driven effects of non-nutritive sweeteners on human glucose tolerance', *Cell* (2022), 185(18), pp. 3,307–28.e19, https://pubmed.ncbi.nlm.nih.gov/35987213/.

p. 68 **presence of artificial sweeteners in our diets might be one of the big drivers of the obesity crisis:** T. Davidson and S. Swithers, 'A Pavlovian approach to the problem of obesity', *International Journal of Obesity* (2004), 28, pp. 933–5, https://doi.org/10.1038/sj.ijo.0802660; S. E. Swithers, 'Artificial sweeteners are not the answer to childhood obesity', *Appetite* (2015), 93, pp. 85–90, doi:10.1016/j.appet.2015.03.027. Professor Swithers' arguments are controversial, and there have been some studies which seem to suggest her findings may not fully extrapolate to humans: https://www.foodnavigator.com/

Article/2015/04/13/Report-and-industry-clash-over-artificial-sweeteners-role-in-childhood-obesity#, as accessed 10 November 2023.

p. 70 **the average person has 'lost about 40 per cent' of the diverse life in our microbiomes:** C. Clutter, 'Disappearance of the Human Microbiota: How We May Be Losing Our Oldest Allies', *American Society for Microbiology*, 8 November 2019, https://asm.org/Articles/2019/November/Disappearance-of-the-Gut-Microbiota-How-We-May-Be, as accessed 1 July 2023.

p. 70 **Eighty per cent of processed food is made up of just four ingredients:** Spector, *The Diet Myth*, p. 94.

p. 70 **processed foods make you eat, on average, 500 calories more every day:** K. Hall et al., 'Ultra-Processed Diets Cause Excess Calorie Intake and Weight Gain: An Inpatient Randomized Controlled Trial of Ad Libitum Food Intake', *Cell Metabolism* (2019), 30(1), pp. 66–77, https://www.cell.com/cell-metabolism/fulltext/S1550-4131(19)30248-7.

p. 71 **Thirty years ago, it took twelve weeks for a factory-farmed chicken to reach its slaughter weight:** https://www.theguardian.com/environment/2016/apr/24/real-cost-of-roast-chicken-animal-welfare-farms, as accessed 6 November 2023.

p. 71 **Broiler chickens are three times higher in fat today than they were when I was born:** https://www.ciwf.org.uk/media/5234769/Nutritional-benefits-of-higher-welfare-animal-products-June-2012.pdf, as accessed 6 November 2023. These are the figures for intensively reared broiler chickens, which constitute the vast majority of chickens we consume, especially in the United States.

p. 71 **the standard factory-farmed turkey now has such an obese chest that it can barely stand up:** Daniel Imhoff, 'Honoring the Food Animals on Your Plate', *Huffington Post* (2011), https://www.huffpost.com/entry/honoring-food-animals-cafos_b_826016, as accessed 6 November 2023.

p. 72 **lambs will rapidly add 30 per cent to their body weight:** Mark Schatzker, *The Dorito Effect: The Surprising New Truth About Food and Flavor* (Simon & Schuster, 2016), p. 80; 'Molasweet palatant boosts lamb growth', All About Feed (blog), 27 May 2008, https://www.allaboutfeed.net/home/molasweet-palatant-boosts-lamb-growth/ (this study was funded by the food industry).

p. 76 **causing one in every seven women to get breast cancer:** 'Breast cancer statistics', Cancer Research UK, https://www.cancerresearchuk.org/health-professional/cancer-statistics/statistics-by-cancer-type/breast-cancer#:~:text=Breast%20cancer%20risk,in%20the%20UK%20are%20preventable, as accessed 1 October 2023.

p. 76 **That wasn't true ten years ago, twenty years ago, let alone two hundred years ago:** 'Since the early 1990s, breast cancer incidence rates have increased by around a sixth (18%) in the UK', according to Breast Cancer UK. 'Breast cancer statistics', Cancer Research UK.

p. 82 **I thought about this more deeply when I read an essay by the Irish journalist Terry Prone:** T. Prone, 'Moral outrage won't halt demand for new weight-loss drug of choice', *Irish Examiner*, 15 May 2023, https://www.irishexaminer.com/opinion/columnists/arid-41138794.html, as accessed 10 October 2023.

CHAPTER 4 LIVING IN AN INFLAMED STATE

p. 86 **As a result of type 2 diabetes, every year more than 120,000 people:** Centers for Disease Control and Prevention, 'National Diabetes Statistics Report – Coexisting Conditions and Complications', 30 September 2022, https://www.cdc.gov/diabetes/data/statistics-report/coexisting-conditions-complications.html, as accessed 12 October 2023. See also Henry Dimbleby with Jemima Lewis, *Ravenous: How to Get Ourselves and Our Planet into Shape* (Profile, 2023), p. 258.

p. 87 **You lose fifteen years of your life:** Max Pemberton told me via email, 'Adolescents/young adults with Type 2 diabetes lose approximately fifteen years from average RLE [remaining life expectancy] and may experience severe, chronic complications of Type 2 diabetes by their forties.' See E. T. Rhodes et al., 'Estimated morbidity and mortality in adolescents and young adults diagnosed with Type 2 diabetes mellitus', *Diabetic Medicine* (2012), 29(4), pp. 453–63, https://onlinelibrary.wiley.com/doi/10.1111/j.1464-5491.2011.03542.x.

p. 87 **An obese man is six times more likely to develop diabetes than a non-obese man:** D. P. Guh et al., 'The incidence of co-morbidities related to obesity and overweight: a systematic review and meta-analysis', *BMC Public Health* (2009), 9(88), https://bmcpublichealth.biomedcentral.com/articles/10.1186/1471-2458-9-88. I first learned about this study in Nadja Hermann, *Conquering Fat Logic* (Scribe, 2019), p. 101.

p. 87 **A scientific overview looking at 2.3 million individuals with type 2 diabetes:** A. Jayedi et al., 'Anthropometric and adiposity indicators and risk of type 2 diabetes: systematic review and dose-response meta-analysis of cohort studies', *BMJ* (2022), 376, https://www.bmj.com/content/376/bmj-2021-067516.

p. 87 **If your BMI is over 35 when you are eighteen years old, you have an over 70 per cent chance of becoming diabetic:** K. M. V. Narayan et al., 'Effect of BMI on Lifetime Risk for Diabetes in the U.S.', *Diabetes Care*, 1 June 2007, 30(6), pp. 1,562–6, https://doi.org/10.2337/dc06-2544.

p. 87 **In a simple experiment, a team of scientists took six healthy men:** G. Boden et al., 'Excessive caloric intake acutely causes oxidative stress, GLUT4 carbonylation, and insulin resistance in healthy men', *Science Translational Medicine* (2015), 7(304), p. 304re7, doi:10.1126/scitranslmed.aac4765. I first learned about this study in Rachel Herz, *Why You Eat What You Eat* (W. W. Norton & Co., 2019), pp. 12–13.

p. 87 **more than a third of the US population is currently in a pre-diabetic state:** A. Menke, S. Casagrande, L. Geiss and C. C. Cowie, 'Prevalence of and Trends in Diabetes Among Adults in the United States, 1988–2012', *JAMA* (2015), 314(10), pp. 1,021–29, doi: 10.1001/jama.2015.10029. I first learned about this study in Hermann, *Conquering Fat Logic*, p. 100. See also the CDC website, which estimates 96 million American adults have prediabetes, 'more than 1 in 3': https://www.cdc.gov/chronicdisease/resources/publications/factsheets/diabetes-prediabetes.htm, as accessed 24 August 2023.

p. 88 **if you're an overweight man, you are 176 per cent more likely:** D. P. Guh et al., 'The incidence of co-morbidities related to obesity and weight: a systematic review and meta-analysis', *BMC Public Health* (2009), 9(88), doi: 10.11.1186/1471-2458-9-88. I first learned about this study in Hermann, *Conquering Fat Logic*, p. 109.

p. 89 **the number of Americans whose death from heart disease was attributed by doctors to obesity:** https://www.washingtonpost.com/wellness/2023/09/18/obesity-heart-disease-cardiac-death/, as accessed 10 October 2023.

p. 89 **greater probability of an ischemic stroke compared with normal-weight subjects:** P. Strazzullo et al., 'Excess Body Weight and Incidence of Stroke: Meta-Analysis of Prospective Studies With 2 Million Participants', *Stroke* (2010), 41(5), e418–e426, https://doi.org/10.1161/STROKEAHA.109.576967. A different recent meta-analysis, using different statistical techniques, found associations between obesity and Type 2 diabetes and obesity and coronary artery disease, but not with stroke: H. Riaz et al., 'Association Between Obesity and Cardiovascular Outcomes: A Systematic Review and Meta-analysis of Mendelian Randomization Studies', *JAMA Network Open* (2018), 1(7), e183788, doi:10.1001/jamanetworkopen.2018.3788.

p. 90 **between 4 and 8 per cent of cancers are attributable to obesity:** S. Pati et al., 'Obesity and Cancer: A Current Overview of Epidemiology, Pathogenesis, Outcomes, and Management', *Cancers (Basel)* (2023), 15, 2, p. 485, https://www.ncbi.nlm.nih.gov/pmc/articles/PMC9857053/; https://www.cancerresearchuk.org/about-cancer/causes-of-cancer/obesity-weight-and-cancer#:~:text=Overweight%20and%20obesity%20is%20the,you%20are%20a%20healthy%20weight, as accessed 28 October 2023.

p. 90 **linking obesity to not just one but nine different types of cancer:** K. Kelland, 'Fat to blame for half a million cancers a year', *Reuters*, 25 November 2014, https://www.scientificamerican.com/article/fat-to-blame-for-half-a-million-cancers-a-year/, as accessed 2 July 2023; M. Kyrgiou et al., 'Adiposity and cancer at major anatomical sites: umbrella review of the literature', *BMJ* (2017), 356, j477, https://www.bmj.com/content/356/bmj.j477.

p. 90 **The leading British cancer charity, Cancer Research UK, explains:** 'How does obesity cause cancer?', Cancer Research UK, 14 February 2023, https://www.cancerresearchuk.org/about-cancer/causes-of-cancer/bodyweight-and-cancer/how-does-obesity-cause-cancer, as accessed 14 October 2023.

p. 92 **The findings are startling:** T. D. Adams et al., 'Long-Term Mortality after Gastric Bypass Surgery', *New England Journal of Medicine* (2007), 357, pp. 753–61, https://www.nejm.org/doi/full/10.1056/nejmoa066603, as cited in *Oxford Handbook*, p. 797; R. Khamsi, 'Stomach stapling really can save lives', *New Scientist*, 22 August 2007, https://www.newscientist.com/article/dn12526-stomach-stapling-really-can-save-lives/#:~:text=They%20found%20that%20within%20about,overall%20reduced%20risk%20of%20death, as accessed 3 August 2023. See also J. Radcliffe, *Cut Down to Size: Achieving Success with Weight Loss Surgery* (Routledge, 2013), pp. 150–2; Hermann, *Conquering Fat Logic*, p. 116.

p. 93 **the results of the first major study into how using Wegovy:** H. Kuchler, 'Weight-loss drugs: will health systems and insurers pay for "skinny jabs"?', *Financial Times*, 11 August 2023, https://www.ft.com/content/81ca6f61-b945-4975-95ff-23ad0a4d8faa, as accessed 13 August 2023.

p. 94 **we could prevent one in five of the heart attacks or strokes:** N. D. Wong et al., 'US Population Eligibility and Estimated Impact of Semaglutide Treatment on Obesity Prevalence and Cardiovascular Disease Events', *Cardiovascular Drugs and Therapy* (2023), https://doi.org/10.1007/s10557-023-07488-3.

CHAPTER 5 AN OLD STORY REPEATING ITSELF?

p. 98 **much more likely to experience paranoia, anxiety, psychosis and damage to your heart:** Alicia Mundy, *Dispensing With the Truth* (St Martin's Press, 2001), p. 38.

p. 101 **Mary Linnen was a typical person taking the drug:** Ibid., pp. 1–8.

announced 'a thyroid cancer safety signal' for all GLP-1 agonists: N. Skydsgaard, 'Novo Nordisk says EMA raised safety signal on drugs including semaglutide', *Reuters*, 22 June 2023, https://www.reuters.com/business/healthcare-pharmaceuticals/novo-nordisk-shares-slip-ema-drug-safety-signal-2023-06-22/.

p. 106 **when GLP-1 agonists are given to rats and mice:** M. A. Nauck and N. Friedrich, 'Do GLP-1-based therapies increase cancer risk?', *Diabetes Care* (2013), 36, suppl. 2, S245–52, https://www.ncbi.nlm.nih.gov/pmc/articles/PMC3920789/#B6; L. B. Knudsen et al., 'Glucagon-Like

Peptide-1 Receptor Agonists Activate Rodent Thyroid C-Cells Causing Calcitonin Release and C-Cell Proliferation', *Endocrinology* (2010), 151(4), pp. 1,473–86, https://doi.org/10.1210/en.2009-1272 https://pubmed.ncbi.nlm.nih.gov/20203154/.

p. 107 **Their findings were startling:** J. Bezin et al., 'GLP-1 Receptor Agonists and the Risk of Thyroid Cancer', *Diabetes Care* (2023), 46(2), pp. 384–90, https://diabetesjournals.org/care/article/46/5/e120/148795/Comment-on-Bezin-et-al-GLP-1-Receptor-Agonists-and.

p. 108 **a very slight chance of a condition named pancreatitis:** S. Singh et al., 'Glucagonlike Peptide 1-Based Therapies and Risk of Hospitalization for Acute Pancreatitis in Type 2 Diabetes Mellitus: A Population-Based Matched Case-Control Study', *JAMA Internal Medicine* (2013), 173(7), pp. 534–9, https://jamanetwork.com/journals/jamainternalmedicine/fullarticle/1656537.

p. 109 **analysed health data for people taking semaglutide (Ozempic and Wegovy):** M. Sodhi et al., 'Risk of Gastrointestinal Adverse Events Associated With Glucagon-Like Peptide-1 Receptor Agonists for Weight Loss', *JAMA*, published online 5 October 2023, https://jamanetwork.com/journals/jama/fullarticle/2810542. See also Thomson Reuters, 'New study ties weight-loss drugs Wegovy, Ozempic to serious gastrointestinal conditions', CBC, 5 October 2023, https://www.cbc.ca/news/health/ozempic-wegovy-glp-1-1.6988122#:~:text=Medicines%20in%20the%20same%20class,obesity%20drug%2C%20Canadian%20researchers%20find.

p. 110 **Brea Hand (who isn't involved in the court case) told CBS News:** S. Moniuszko, 'Ozempic, Mounjaro manufacturers sued over claims of "stomach paralysis" side effects', 3 August 2023, https://www.cbsnews.com/news/ozempic-mounjaro-lawsuit-gastroparesis-stomach-paralysis-side-effect/, as accessed 10 October 2023.

Novo Nordisk – who make Ozempic and Wegovy – sent a detailed response, which you can read in full in the extended endnotes: I put the following questions to Novo Nordisk:

Dear Novo Nordisk media team,

I am a British journalist who has written a book which is being published by Bloomsbury Publishing in the UK and Crown Publishing in the US about the new weight loss drugs and their implications. There is information about me at www.johannhari.com. It is a balanced book investigating both the significant health advantages of these drugs (which I myself am taking, and benefitting from) and the potential risks. I am looking at this matter from a personal, human and scientific perspective.

I am writing to you to give you the right of reply and an opportunity to comment on the potential risks/drawbacks of these drugs that I will be raising in the book in respect of GLP-1 agonists.

Please could you respond with any comments on the below statements by Tuesday November 21st:

1. If a user stops taking Ozempic, Wegovy or other GLP-1 agonists, the user on average regains two-thirds of the weight they lost when on GLP-1 agonists within twelve months as shown for example in this study:

Wilding, JPH, Batterham, RL, Davies, M, et al. *Weight regain and cardiometabolic effects after withdrawal of semaglutide: The STEP 1 trial extension. Diabetes Obes Metab.* 2022; 24(8): 1553-1564. doi:10.1111/dom.14725

2. The longer term risks to health from Ozempic, Wegovy or other GLP-1 agonists are not known and so there could be serious negative health effects for some users. For example, anti-psychotics were first developed in the 1950s, but the fact they cause dementia only became clear 50 years later:

Jonas, K., Abi-Dargham, A., & Kotov, R. (2021). *Two hypotheses on the high incidence of dementia in psychotic disorders. JAMA Psychiatry*. Published online September 15, 2021. doi:10.1001/jamapsychiatry.2021.2584 (Link).

I am not suggesting GLP-1 agonists cause dementia – only that they may have presently unknown long-term effects.

3. One longer term effect of Ozempic, Wegovy or other GLP-1 agonists could be damage to children in the womb, where the mother has taken GLP-1 agonists during pregnancy, such that their brain development could be negatively impaired and could lead to increased risk of impaired reward responses, impulsivity, attentional issues, autism or predisposition to substance abuse:

Warning labels on these drugs advise women not to take them whilst pregnant – "may harm your unborn baby", "may cause foetal harm". Animal studies have indicated there may be risks to neonatal development, and no good human studies exist:

See: https://www.ozempic.com; https://www.wegovy.com/taking-wegovy/how-to-use-the-wegovy-pen.html; https://www.accessdata.fda.gov/drugsatfda_docs/label/2022/215866s000lbl.pdf

For more detailed information see:

https://www.drugwatch.com/news/2023/09/07/fda-warning-pregnancy-wegovy-ozempic/amp/

"Studies in pregnant rats have shown embryofoetal mortality, structural abnormalities, and alterations to growth when administered during organogenesis at maternal exposures below the maximum recommended human dose (MRHD). Early pregnancy losses and structural abnormalities were observed in rabbits at doses below the MRHD. In cynomolgus monkeys, early pregnancy losses and structural abnormalities were observed at exposures of 10-fold or higher that of the MRHD. In rabbits and monkeys, these finding coincided with marked maternal body weight loss. Salcaprozate sodium (SNAC), an absorption enhancer in the oral tablet has been shown to cross the placenta and reach fetal tissue in rats. Administration of SNAC to pregnant rats has shown an increase in number of stillbirths and a decrease in pup viability. There are no adequate and well-controlled studies in pregnant women." From https://www.drugs.com/pregnancy/semaglutide.html

These concerns about neonatal development in humans were raised with me by reputable scientists in the field.

4. Ozempic, Wegovy or other GLP-1 agonists increase the risk of contracting thyroid cancer. For instance, French scientists found that GLP-1 agonists increase an individual's risk of thyroid cancer by 58 percent from what it would have been had they not taken the drug: https://diabetesjournals.org/care/article-abstract/46/2/384/147888/GLP-1-Receptor-Agonists-and-the-Risk-of-Thyroid?redirectedFrom=fulltext.

Julien Bezin, Amandine Gouverneur, Marine Pénichon, Clément Mathieu, Renaud Garrel, Dominique Hillaire-Buys, Antoine Pariente, Jean-Luc Faillie; *GLP-1 Receptor Agonists and the Risk of Thyroid Cancer. Diabetes Care* 1 February 2023; 46 (2): 384–390. https://doi.org/10.2337/dc22-1148

https://diabetesjournals.org/care/article-abstract/46/2/384/147888/GLP-1-Receptor-Agonists-and-the-Risk-of-Thyroid?redirectedFrom=fulltext

This was a study using statistical methods to estimate any increased risk of thyroid cancer found in diabetics taking GLP-1 receptor agonists between 2006 and 2018. They were matched with "control" diabetics who were not taking the drugs. The analysis attempted to control for various factors including whether or not patients were taking any other antidiabetes drugs and relative levels of socioeconomic deprivation. After controlling for these they still found substantial increased risks.

The 58% increased risk is the estimate for all thyroid cancers; they found a 78% increased risk of medullary thyroid cancer in particular.

5. Ozempic, Wegovy or other GLP-1 agonists increase the risk of pancreatitis and stomach paralysis and bowel obstruction, which in some cases will result in a user's organ failure and death. For instance, Canadian scientists found that GLP-1 agonists significantly increase the risks of pancreatitis and stomach paralysis:

https://jamanetwork.com/journals/jama/fullarticle/2810542. Sodhi M, Rezaeianzadeh R, Kezouh A, Etminan M. *Risk of Gastrointestinal Adverse Events Associated With Glucagon-Like Peptide-1 Receptor Agonists for Weight Loss. JAMA*. Published online October 05, 2023. doi:10.1001/jama.2023.19574 https://jamanetwork.com/journals/jama/fullarticle/2810542

Those taking Ozempic, Wegovy or other GLP-1 agonists were nine times more likely than those taking a different anti-obesity drug to get pancreatitis, and more than three and a half times more likely to get gastroparesis (stomach paralysis). That's a 909% increased risk of pancreatitis and a 367% increased risk of gastroparesis.

6. That, like other forms of weight loss, the loss caused by Ozempic, Wegovy or other GLP-1 agonists can cause a loss of muscle mass and

sarcopenia, which can have negative health effects, especially for older people as it can lead to falls and death:

This issue is widely discussed in relation to GLP-1 agonists, and pharmaceutical companies are currently investigating ways to mitigate this risk, see:

M. Lenharo, "Anti-obesity drugs' side effects: what we know so far", *Nature* 622, 682 (2023) https://www.nature.com/articles/d41586-023-03183-3

There is evidence that a higher BMI may be protective as we age and/or that losing too much weight later in life isn't necessarily a good thing, in part for this reason. See for example:

Associations of Change in Body Size With All-Cause and Cause-Specific Mortality Among Healthy Older Adults, 2023; "This study suggests that weight loss was associated with an increase in mortality, particularly among men, highlighting the need to monitor and investigate weight loss in older adults."

Body mass index and all-cause mortality in older adults: A scoping review of observational studies, 2020; "Overweight BMI classification or a higher BMI value may be protective with regard to all-cause mortality, relative to normal BMI, in older adults. These findings demonstrate the potential need for age-specific BMI cut-points in older adults."

The Influence of Age the BMI and All-Cause Mortality Association: A Meta-Analysis, 2017; "The recommended healthy weight range is appropriate for younger and middle aged adults but a higher BMI range should be recommended for older adults based on mortality."

7. That a small minority of people taking these drugs may experience malnutrition as a result:

This issue is widely discussed in relation to Ozempic, Wegovy or other GLP-1 agonists, see for example:

https://www.nytimes.com/2023/04/21/well/eat/ozempic-side-effects-malnutrition.html which includes quotes from Dr. Andrew Kraftson, a clinical associate professor in the division of metabolism, endocrinology and diabetes at Michigan Medicine, who prescribes diets to patients whom he puts on these drugs, hoping to ensure they eat a minimum level of calories.

8. That since these drugs seem to have positive effects on the brain, leading people to want to over-eat less, that there is the possibility that they also have negative effects on the brain, so that use of GLP-1 agonists may in the future be confirmed to cause harm to brain function:

Evidence that the drugs work on the brain's reward system is extremely strong and well-accepted, see for example:

Turton MD, O'Shea D, Gunn I, et al. 'A role for glucagon-like peptide-1 in the central regulation of feeding'. *Nature*. 1996;379(6560):69-72. doi:10.1038/379069a0

Jerlhag E. 'The therapeutic potential of glucagon-like peptide-1 for persons with addictions based on findings from preclinical and clinical studies'. *Front*

Pharmacol. 2023 Mar 30;14:1063033. doi: 10.3389/fphar.2023.1063033. PMID: 37063267; PMCID: PMC10097922.

Tufvesson-Alm M, Shevchouk OT, Jerlhag E. 'Insight into the role of the gut-brain axis in alcohol-related responses: Emphasis on GLP-1, amylin, and ghrelin'. *Front Psychiatry*. 2023 Jan 9;13:1092828. doi: 10.3389/fpsyt.2022.1092828. PMID: 36699502; PMCID: PMC9868418.

Aranäs C, Edvardsson CE, Shevchouk OT, Zhang Q, Witley S, Blid Sköldheden S, Zentveld L, Vallöf D, Tufvesson-Alm M, Jerlhag E. 'Semaglutide reduces alcohol intake and relapse-like drinking in male and female rats'. *EBioMedicine*. 2023 Jul;93:104642. doi: 10.1016/j.ebiom.2023.104642. Epub 2023 Jun 7. PMID: 37295046; PMCID: PMC10363436.

Douton, JE, Horvath, N, Mills-Huffnagle, S, Nyland, JE, Hajnal, A, Grigson, PS. 'Glucagon-like peptide-1 receptor agonist, liraglutide, reduces heroin self-administration and drug-induced reinstatement of heroin-seeking behaviour in rats'. *Addiction Biology*. 2022; 27(2):e13117. doi:10.1111/adb.13117

These concerns were raised to me when I interviewed many reputable scientists in the field.

9. Such harm to brain function as mentioned above may result in anhedonia or increased depression. Such harm to brain function as mentioned above may be related to the safety signal raised around suicide in relation to these drugs:

Brain effects are being actively explored for positive impact, but where there is impact there is always the risk of negative impacts also.

This 2023 online interview with an American researcher who is currently investigating semaglutide in relation to alcoholism makes it clear that anhedonia is widely discussed as a possible risk: https://news.okstate.edu/articles/health-sciences/2023/osu-chs-researcher-studying-weight-loss-drugs-alcohol-use-disorder-treatment.html

The European Medicines Agency released this press statement in July 2023 about the suicide safety signal which was raised by Icelandic doctors in relation to GLP-1 agonists: https://www.ema.europa.eu/en/news/ema-statement-ongoing-review-glp-1-receptor-agonists

These concerns were raised to me when I interviewed many reputable scientists in the field.

10. Even if Ozempic, Wegovy or other GLP-1 agonists are taken indefinitely, there are grounds to suspect that increasing tolerance or physiological and neural change may render the drug ineffective at weight control over time:

As the drugs are so newly-approved for treating obesity, it is hard to point to long-term studies indicating tolerance effects. However the rate of weight loss in the clinical trials seems to level off after several months on semaglutide, and there is an indication that weight may even be beginning to be regained at the end of the longest trial, STEP One: body weight change reached its nadir at week 60, with a slight uptick visible in the final 8 weeks on treatment. See Table 1 in: https://www.nejm.org/doi/full/10.1056/NEJMoa2032183

Interviews within my book make it clear that tolerance is well-known as a likely issue with long-term use of drugs.

See also: https://www.msdmanuals.com/en-gb/home/drugs/factors-affecting-response-to-drugs/tolerance-and-resistance-to-drugs

11. Use of Ozempic, Wegovy or other GLP-1 agonists might result in such loss of pleasure from eating for some people, that harmful habits may take hold as some users may seek stimulation and pleasure in other ways, which may be personally and socially harmful.

This side effect is widely reported, and many of my own interviewees referred to it. See also, for example, patients interviewed in this article: https://www.nytimes.com/2023/04/21/well/eat/ozempic-side-effects-malnutrition.html

12. Despite the fact there is guidance given for Ozempic, Wegovy or other GLP-1 agonists that they should not be given to people with a BMI lower than 27, some people with eating disorders who are highly motivated to deprive themselves of food may get hold of these drugs (mainly through online prescriptions) and harm themselves as a result. This risk is being widely discussed:

UK eating disorders charity, Beat, issued this press release 8 March 2023, when Wegovy was approved by the NHS, saying that semaglutide is "very dangerous for those with eating disorders": https://www.beateatingdisorders.org.uk/news/semaglutide-weight-loss-medication-very-dangerous-for-those-with-eating-disorders/

In the same month UK pharmacist Superdrug was cautioned for advertising the drug online – see reporting in the *Guardian*: https://www.theguardian.com/society/2023/mar/12/explainer-new-skinny-jab-has-been-approved-by-the-nhs-but-does-it-work-and-can-you-buy-it

And the Chair of the eating disorder faculty at the Royal College of Psychiatrists was quoted as saying these drugs pose "a real danger for abuse of the medication by those for whom there is no clinical need to use it": https://www.independent.co.uk/news/health/nhs-weight-loss-jab-eating-disorders-b2296680.html

These issues were raised with me by some of the leading experts on eating disorders in the United States.

Please do let me know if you would like to make any other comments about Ozempic, Wegovy or other GLP-1 agonists. In the book in addition to discussing these potential risks I also discuss many benefits of the drugs.

I received the following reply from their spokesperson.

Our Response, attributable to a Novo Nordisk spokesperson:

Patient safety is paramount to Novo Nordisk, and we work closely with national health authorities to continuously monitor the safety profile of our medicines.

GLP-1 RAs have been used to treat type 2 diabetes for more than 15 years, and for the treatment of obesity for 8 years, including Novo Nordisk medicines that have been on the market for more than 10 years. Semaglutide has been examined in large global clinical development programs, and real-world evidence studies. Cumulatively it has over 12 million patient years of exposure.[i]

Treatment decisions should be made together with a healthcare provider who can evaluate the appropriateness of using a GLP-1 RA medicine based on assessment of a patient's individual medical profile and in accordance with the medicine Summary of Product Characteristics.

Additional Information on background

Please note that for any questions not directly referenced below, we would refer you to the above statement.

Please note that we have reason to feel that your book may be listed on Bloomsbury with working title "The Magic Pill". If this is the case please note that Ozempic/Wegovy are available as subcutaneous injections and not as oral formulations or pills. If the use of pill in the title is intended to refer to Wegovy or Ozempic we would flag that "magic pill" is an inaccurate characterisation of these medicines and the title should be updated.

Indications

Please note the indications for our semaglutide products.

UK indications

Ozempic® ▼ (semaglutide injection) is indicated for the treatment of adults with insufficiently controlled type 2 diabetes mellitus as an adjunct to diet and exercise. Ozempic® is not licensed for the treatment of weight management.[ii]

Rybelsus ▼ (semaglutide tablets) is indicated for the treatment of adults with insufficiently controlled type 2 diabetes mellitus to improve glycaemic control as an adjunct to diet and exercise. Rybelsus® is not licensed for the treatment of weight management.[iii]

Wegovy® ▼ (semaglutide injection) is indicated as an adjunct to a reduced-calorie diet and increased physical activity for weight management, including weight loss and weight maintenance, in adults with an initial Body Mass Index (BMI) of

≥30 kg/m2 (obesity), or ≥27 kg/m2 to <30 kg/m2 (overweight) in the presence of at least one weight-related comorbidity.[iv]

U.S. Indications

Ozempic® (semaglutide) is FDA-approved for the treatment of type 2 diabetes, to improve blood sugar, along with diet and exercise, and reduce the risk of major cardiovascular events such as heart attack, stroke, or death in adults with type 2 diabetes and known heart disease. Ozempic® is not approved for chronic weight management. Please see Ozempic® full prescribing information here.

Rybelsus® (semaglutide) tablets is FDA-approved for the treatment of type 2 diabetes, to improve blood sugar, along with diet and exercise in adults with type 2 diabetes. It was clinically researched and studied in patients with type 2 diabetes. Rybelsus® is not approved for chronic weight management. Please see Rybelsus® full prescribing information here.

Wegovy® (semaglutide) is FDA-approved for chronic weight management in adults with obesity (BMI > 30), or overweight (excess weight) (BMI > 27) who also have weight-related medical problems, used with a reduced-calorie meal plan and increased physical activity. Wegovy® is also indicated for use in patients aged 12 years and older with an initial BMI at or above the 95th percentile for age and sex. Please see Wegovy® full prescribing information here.

NOTE: Although Wegovy®, Ozempic® and Rybelsus® all contain semaglutide, they are different products with different indications, dosages, prescribing information, titration schedules, and delivery forms. The products are not interchangeable and should not be used outside of their approved indications. Novo Nordisk is committed to the responsible use of our medicines and is taking multiple steps to ensure responsible use of our semaglutide medicines which are detailed on semaglutide.com.

Re: Question 1 on weight regain.

Results from the STEP trials demonstrate that weight regain is likely once treatment with Wegovy® is stopped. Clinical experts consulted by Novo Nordisk view obesity as a chronic disease that should be managed similar to other long-term health conditions such as diabetes and hypertension.[v]

NOTE: Please note that the Wilding reference you have shared is with regards to Wegovy® specifically and not other GLP-1 receptor agonists.

Re: Question 3 on any effect of GLP-1 Ras on unborn children during pregnancy.

The Summary of Product Characteristics (SmPC) for our semaglutide medicines state that these medicines should not be used during pregnancy. [ii], [iii], [iv] We recommend patients take semaglutide only for its approved indications and under the supervision of a healthcare professional.

Pregnancy or intention to become pregnant were exclusion criteria in our trials with semaglutide in both obesity and type 2 diabetes. There are therefore limited clinical trial data with semaglutide use in pregnant women. However, in the U.S., information related to pregnancy appears in Section 8.1 & 8.3 of the U.S. Prescribing Information for both Ozempic® and Wegovy®.

There is an ongoing study to evaluate the safety of exposure to Wegovy® during pregnancy on Clinical Trials.govhere: https://classic.clinicaltrials.gov/ct2/show/NCT05503927

Re: Question 4 on any risk of contracting thyroid cancer from GLP-1 medicines.

Recently the European Medicines Agency has conducted an independent investigation into any association between GLP-1 RA medicines (note: as a class, not only our medicines) and risk of thyroid cancer. On 27th October 2023, the EMA found no causal association between the GLP-1 RAs, namely – exenatide, liraglutide, dulaglutide, semaglutide, and lixisenatide – and cancer of the thyroid.[vi]

Re: Question 5 on acute pancreatitis and gastroparesis. Gastrointestinal (GI) events are common side effects of the GLP-1 class. For semaglutide, most GI side effects were mild to moderate in severity and of short duration. [ii], [iii], [iv] GLP-1RAs are known to effect a delay in gastric emptying, as detailed in the Summary of Product Characteristics (SmPC). [ii], [iii], [iv] Acute Pancreatitis, is also listed as an adverse reaction in the SMPC. [ii], [iii], [iv]

The long-term data from SELECT published recently with Semaglutide exposure over 39 months is reassuring that there is no increase in the risk of pancreatitis with Semaglutide 2.4 in comparison with placebo.

Re: Question 6 on any effect of semaglutide on body composition (including fat mass and lean mass).

In clinical trials for Wegovy®, Ozempic® or Rybelsus®, we did not specifically study the medicine's impact on muscle mass. In a sub-study of 140 patients with a BMI of 40 or less conducted as part of the STEP 1 trial, dual-energy x-ray absorptiometry (DEXA) analyses suggested that treatment with Wegovy® was accompanied by reductions in both fat mass and lean body mass, with a greater reduction in fat mass than lean body mass. We recommend that any patients experiencing side effects while taking Wegovy®, Ozempic® or Rybelsus® contact their healthcare provider.

Re: Question 9 on any risk of suicidal ideation.

Novo Nordisk will continue to monitor reports of adverse drug reactions, including suicide and suicidal ideation, through routine pharmacovigilance and in cooperation with local health authorities.

In the U.S., FDA requires medications for chronic weight management that work on the central nervous system, including Wegovy® and Saxenda®, to carry a warning about suicidal behavior and ideation. This event had been reported in clinical trials with other weight management products. Novo Nordisk is continuously performing surveillance of the data from ongoing clinical trials and real-world use of its products and collaborates closely with the authorities to ensure patient safety and adequate information to healthcare professionals. Novo Nordisk remains confident in the benefit risk profile of the products and remains committed to ensuring patient safety.

The long term data from SELECT published recently with Semaglutide exposure over 39 months is reassuring that there is no increase in the risk of psychiatric disorders with Semaglutide 2.4 in comparison with placebo.

Re: Question 12 on potential use of GLP-1 RAs by people living with eating disorders.

Novo Nordisk does not promote, suggest, or encourage off-label use, or misuse, or any of our medications. We do our best to ensure patients and doctors are educated about the appropriate use of our products and encourage healthcare providers to only prescribe the right product for the right patient.

Novo Nordisk is committed to the responsible use of our medicines and is taking multiple steps to ensure responsible use of our semaglutide medicines which for people living in the US are detailed on semaglutide.com.

References

[i] Novo Nordisk A/S. Semaglutide PSUR/PBRER dated 18 July 2023, Version 1.0 (01 Jun 2022–31 May 2023). Data on file.

[ii] Ozempic® SMPC. Available at: https://www.ema.europa.eu/en/documents/product-information/ozempic-epar-product-information_en.pdf [Last Accessed November 2023].

[iii] Rybelsus® SMPC. Available at: https://www.ema.europa.eu/en/documents/product-information/rybelsus-epar-product-information_en.pdf [Last Accessed November 2023].

[iv] Wegovy® SMPC. Available at: https://www.ema.europa.eu/en/documents/product-information/wegovy-epar-product-information_en.pdf [Last Accessed November 2023].

[v] Novo Nordisk. Data on file.

[vi] Meeting highlights from the Pharmacovigilance Risk Assessment Committee (PRAC) 23-26 October 2023. Available at: https://www.ema.europa.eu/en/news/meeting-highlights-pharmacovigilance-risk-assessment-committee-prac-23-26-october-2023 [Last accessed November 2023]

CHAPTER 6 WHY DON'T YOU DIET AND EXERCISE INSTEAD?

p. 125 **followed dieters rigorously for two years, or, in a few cases, five years:** T. Mann et al., 'Medicare's search for effective obesity treatments: Diets are not the answer', *American Psychologist* (2007), 62, pp. 220–33. See also A. J. Tomiyama, B. Ahlstrom and T. Mann, 'Long-term effects of dieting: Is weight loss related to health?' *Social and Personality Psychology Compass* (2013), 7(12), pp. 861–77.

p. 127 **Michael was convinced that 'we do have a set point':** W. Bennett and J. Gurin, *The Dieter's Dilemma* (Basic Books, 1982). This was one of the earliest books putting forward this idea. See the following for more recent discussion: V. M. Ganipisetti and P. Bollimunta, 'Obesity and Set-Point Theory' (updated 25 April 2023), StatPearls; W. T. Garvey, 'Is Obesity or Adiposity-Based Chronic Disease Curable: The Set Point Theory, the Environment, and Second-Generation Medications', *Endocrine Practice* (2022), 28(2), pp. 214–22, doi:10.1016/j.eprac.2021.11.082.

p. 132 **all the best scientific studies of structured weight-loss programmes in the US:** J. W. Anderson et al., 'Long-term weight-loss maintenance: a meta-analysis of US studies', *American Journal of Clinical Nutrition* (2001), 74(5), pp. 579–84, https://pubmed.ncbi.nlm.nih.gov/11684524/.

p. 132 **Another team at Brown Medical School in Rhode Island surveyed the limited evidence:** R. R. Wing and S. Phelan, 'Long-term weight loss maintenance', *American Journal of Clinical Nutrition* (2005), 82, suppl. 1, pp. 222S–225S, https://pubmed.ncbi.nlm.nih.gov/16002825/.

p. 136 **Icelandic kids are among the fattest on the continent:** This is especially true of Icelandic boys. See p. 12 of this PDF: https://www.who.int/europe/publications/i/item/9789289057738; 'WHO European Regional Obesity Report 2022', World Health Organization, 2 May 2022, https://www.who.int/europe/publications/i/item/9789289057738. See also University of Iceland, 'Obesity among Icelandic children grows fast', undated, https://english.hi.is/obesity_among_icelandic_children_grows_fast; 'Icelandic children are the second fattest in Europe', *Iceland Monitor*, 24 May 2017; https://icelandmonitor.mbl.is/news/politics_and_society/2017/05/24/icelandic_children_are_the_second_fattest_in_europe/.

p. 136 **eighty-one women to walk on a treadmill for half an hour, three times a week:** B. J. Sawyer et al., 'Predictors of fat mass changes in response to aerobic exercise training in women', *Journal of Strength and Conditioning Research* (2015), 29(2), pp. 297–304, https://pubmed.ncbi.nlm.nih.gov/25353081/; Hermann, *Conquering Fat Logic*, p. 246.

p. 136 **only 2 per cent of people who lost 2.2 stone or more:** E. Dolgin, 'The appetite genes: Why some of us are born to eat too much', *New Scientist*, 31 May 2017, https://www.newscientist.com/article/mg23431281-600-the-appetite-genes-why-some-of-us-are-born-to-eat-too-much/.

p. 137 **more likely to develop over forty chronic diseases, from diabetes to colon cancer:** N. Twilley, 'A pill to make exercise obsolete', *The New Yorker*, 30 October 2017, https://www.newyorker.com/magazine/2017/11/06/a-pill-to-make-exercise-obsolete.

p. 137 **If you exercise for 270 hours a year, you'll add, on average, three years to your life:** Tim Spector, *The Diet Myth: The Real Science Behind What We Eat* (Weidenfeld & Nicolson, 2016), p. 37.

CHAPTER 7 THE BRAIN BREAKTHROUGH

p. 142 **It turned out that they actually have receptors for GLP-1 in their brains:** https://www.sciencedirect.com/science/article/abs/pii/000689938 9906288.

p. 144 **Diana discovered that the rats who'd had GLP-1:** M. D. Turton et al., 'A role for glucagon-like peptide-1 in the central regulation of feeding', *Nature* (1996), 379(6560), pp. 69–72, doi:10.1038/379069a0, https://pubmed.ncbi.nlm.nih.gov/8538742/.

p. 146 **So she embarked on a series of experiments to find out:** E. Jerlhag, 'The therapeutic potential of glucagon-like peptide-1 for persons with addictions based on findings from preclinical and clinical studies', *Frontiers in Pharmacology* (30 March 2023), 14, 1063033, doi: 10.3389/fphar.2023.1063033. PMID: 37063267; PMCID: PMC10097922; M. Tufvesson-Alm, O. T. Shevchouk and E. Jerlhag, 'Insight into the role of the gut-brain axis in alcohol-related responses: Emphasis on GLP-1, amylin, and ghrelin', *Frontiers in Psychiatry* (9 January 2023), 13, 1092828, doi: 10.3389/fpsyt.2022.1092828;; C. Aranäs et al., 'Semaglutide reduces alcohol intake and relapse-like drinking in male and female rats', *EBioMedicine* (July 2023), 93, 104642, doi: 10.1016/j.ebiom.2023.104642.

p. 149 **giving GLP-1 agonists to rats cut their use of heroin or fentanyl:** J. E. Douton et al., 'Glucagon-like peptide-1 receptor agonist, liraglutide, reduces heroin self-administration and drug-induced reinstatement of heroin-seeking behaviour in rats', Penn State Neuroscience Institute (2022), doi: 10.1111/adb.13117. As Patricia explained via email: 'The GLP-1R agonists reduced cue-induced opioid seeking again very reliably, by about 50%, and when seeking was elicited by a drug prime (or reminder) opioid seeking was reduced by more than 80%. Douton et al., 2021, doi: 10.1097/FBP.0000000000000609; PMID, 33229892 shows the effect of exendin-4 on cue- and drug-induced heroin seeking; Evans et al., 2022; Evans et al., 2022, doi: 10.1016/j.brainresbull.2022.08.022 shows effect of chronic treatment with the longer acting GLP-1R agonist, liraglutide, on cue- and drug-induced heroin seeking; Douton et al., 2022, doi: 10.1097/FBP.0000000000000685. Epub 2022 Jun 7. PMID, 35695511 shows the effect of acutely administered liraglutide on cue-, drug-, and stress-induced heroin seeking; Urbanik et al. 2022 doi: 10.1016/j.brainresbull.2022.08.023 shows the effect of acute administration of liraglutide on cue- and drug-induced fentanyl seeking.'

p. 149 **A team at Florida State University:** G. Sørensen et al., 'The glucagon-like peptide 1 (GLP-1) receptor agonist exendin-4 reduces cocaine self-administration in mice', *Physiology Behavior* (2015), 149, pp. 262–8, doi:10.1016/j.physbeh.2015.06.013.

p. 152 **So far, it looks like GLP-1 agonists do reduce smoking:** Yammine et al., 2021; Yammine et al., 2023. DOI: 10.1097/ADM.0000000000001147 https://academic.oup.com/ntr/article-abstract/23/10/1682/6217746 See also https://sciencenews.dk/en/weight-loss-drug-shows-potential-in-smoking-cessation.

p. 152 **They do reduce alcohol use – but only in overweight people who had an alcohol problem:** https://doi.org/10.1172/jci.

p. 153 **For example, if you have Parkinson's disease:** D. Weintraub et al., 'Association of dopamine agonist use with impulse control disorders in Parkinson disease', *Archives of Neurology* (2006), 63(7), pp. 969–73, doi:10.1001/archneur.63.7.969; Laura E. De Wit, et al, 'Impulse control disorders associated with dopaminergic drugs: A disproportionality analysis using vigibase', *European Neuropsychopharmacology* (2022), 58, pp. 30–8, ISSN 0924-977X, https://doi.org/10.1016/j.euroneuro.2022.01.113. See also 'The medications that change who we are', BBC, undated, https://www.bbc.com/future/article/20200108-the-medications-that-change-who-we-are, as accessed 13 July 2023.

CHAPTER 8 WHAT JOB WAS OVEREATING DOING FOR YOU?

p. 167 **scientists analysed 475 games from the 2004–5 National Football League season:** Herz, *Why You Eat What You Eat*, pp. 247–8, citing Y. Cornil et al., 'From Fan to Fat? Vicarious Losing Increases Unhealthy Eating, but Self-Affirmation Is an Effective Remedy', *Psychological Science* (2013), 24(10), pp. 1,936–46, https://doi.org/10.1177/0956797613481232.

p. 168 **On the night Donald Trump was elected President in 2016:** V. Chamlee, 'On election night, Americans self-medicated with delivery food and booze', *Eater*, 14 November 2016, https://www.eater.com/2016/11/14/13621652/election-night-food-postmates-grubhub; M. LaMagna, 'Here are the comfort foods America binged on as the election unfolded', MarketWatch, 16 November 2016, https://www.marketwatch.com/story/this-is-what-americans-ate-on-election-day-and-after-2016-11-11, as cited in Herz, *Why You Eat What You Eat*, pp. 234–5.

p. 168 **if you lose your job, your chances of adding 10 per cent or more of your body weight shoot up too:** J. K. Morris et al., 'Non-employment and changes in smoking, drinking, and body weight', *BMJ* (1992), 304(6826), pp. 536–41, https://pubmed.ncbi.nlm.nih.gov/1559056/; I first learned about this in Esther Rothblum and Sondra Solovay, eds, *The Fat Studies Reader* (NYU Press, 2009), p. 26.

p. 169 **Among American soldiers who fought in the Vietnam War:** Michael Moss, *Hooked: How We Became Addicted to Processed Food* (W. H. Allen, 2022), p. 70, citing W. V. R. Vieweg et al., 'Body mass index relates to males with posttraumatic stress disorder', *Journal of the*

National Medical Association (2006), 98(4), pp. 580–6, https://www.ncbi.nlm.nih.gov/pmc/articles/PMC2569214/.

p. 171 **there was something going on in the psyches of people who overeat:** For this section about Hilde, I have drawn on a range of sources, particularly Hilde's excellent book *Eating Disorders*. See also Gilman, *Obesity: The Biography*, pp. 94–105; Ellen Ruppel Shell, *The Hungry Gene: The Inside Story of the Obesity Industry* (Grove Press, 2003), pp. 44–5; Rothblum and Solovay, *The Fat Studies Reader*, pp. 114–17; Virginia Sole-Smith, *Fat Talk: Coming of Age in Diet Culture* (Ithaka, 2023), pp. 9, 152; Amy Erdman Farrell, *Fat Shame: Stigma and the Fat Body in American Culture* (NYU Press, 2011), pp. 77–80; *Oxford Handbook*, p. 89.

p. 175 **her team at Penn State Children's Hospital took a group of 279 first-time mothers:** I. M. Paul et al., 'Effect of a Responsive Parenting Educational Intervention on Childhood Weight Outcomes at 3 Years of Age: The INSIGHT Randomized Clinical Trial', *JAMA* (2018), 320(5), pp. 461–8, doi:10.1001/jama.2018.9432.

p. 176 **explore how it helped me to think about these new drugs:** Hari, *Lost Connections*, Chapter 9.

p. 178 **The writer Roxane Gay writes about this in her moving memoir:** I quote here from Roxane Gay, *Hunger: A Memoir of (My) Body* (Harper, 2017), pp. 11 and 142–3.

p. 181 **Roughly one in ten of the people who have bariatric surgery develop an addiction:** J. E. Mitchell et al., 'Addictive disorders after Roux-en-Y gastric bypass', *Integrated Health* (2015), 11, 14, https://doi.org/10.1016/j.soard.2014.10.026. Many of them had had addictions in the past, which were now reactivated.

p. 184 **a significant minority – 17 per cent – experience depression and anxiety:** Mitchell and de Zwaan, Bariatric Surgery, p. 103: 'Powers et al (1992) reported that 17 percent of patients experienced significant psychiatric symptoms postsurgically that required hospitalisation. Mitchell et al (2001) found that 29 percent of their sample experienced an episode of major depression post surgically.' P. S. Powers et al., 'Psychiatric Issues in Bariatric Surgery', *Obesity Surgery* (1992), 2(4), pp. 315–25, https://pubmed.ncbi.nlm.nih.gov/10765191/; J. E. Mitchell et al., 'Long-term follow-up of patients' status after gastric bypass', *Obesity Surgery* (2001), 11(4), pp. 464–8, https://pubmed.ncbi.nlm.nih.gov/11501356/.

p. 184 **After bariatric surgery, we [see an] increase [in] suicide fourfold:** It varies by procedure, and is almost fourfold for gastric bypass, while for others, it is lower. The overall adjusted hazard ratio for suicide after all bariatric surgery is 3.16. See https://www.ncbi.nlm.nih.gov/pmc/articles/PMC5932484/. See also C. Peterhansel et al., 'Risk of completed suicide after bariatric surgery: a systematic review', *Obesity*

Reviews (2013), 14(5), pp. 369–82, https://pubmed.ncbi.nlm.nih.gov/23297762/; D. Castaneda et al., 'Risk of Suicide and Self-harm Is Increased After Bariatric Surgery – A Systematic Review and Meta-analysis', *Obesity Surgery* (2019), 29(1), pp. 322–33, https://pubmed.ncbi.nlm.nih.gov/30343409/.

CHAPTER 9 'I DON'T THINK YOU'RE IN YOUR BODY'

p. 188 **In one study of the effects of Ozempic on weight:** See Figure 1 in J. P. H. Wilding et al., 'Once-Weekly Semaglutide in Adults with Overweight or Obesity', *New England Journal of Medicine* (2021), 384(11), pp. 989–1,002, doi:10.1056/NEJMoa2032183.

p. 197 **Research in the 1950s found that very few people were unhappy with their bodies:** T. F. Cash and L. Smolak (2011), 'Understanding body images: Historical and contemporary perspectives', in T. F. Cash and L. Smolak, eds, *Body Image: A Handbook of Science, Practice, and Prevention* (Guilford Press, 2012), pp. 3–11.

p. 197 **upwards of 90 per cent of women feel some aspect of negative body image:** V. Swami et al., 'Associations between women's body image and happiness: Results of the YouBeauty.com Body Image Survey (YBIS)', *Journal of Happiness Studies* (2015), 16, pp. 705–16. See also https://www.psychologytoday.com/us/articles/199702/body-image-in-america-survey-results, as accessed 6 November 2023.

p. 198 **It tells you you are incomplete:** V. Swami, 'Cross-cultural perspectives on body size', in M. L. Craig, ed., *The Routledge Companion to Beauty Politics* (Routledge, 2023), pp. 103–11.

p. 198 **Then, on social media, we reinforce these ideas:** S. Stieger et al., 'Engagement with social media content results in negative body image: An experience sampling study using wearables and a physical analogue scale', *Body Image* (2022), 43, pp. 232–43.

p. 199 **One group of scientists gathered a hundred people:** B. M. Dolan, S. A. Birtchnell and J. H. Lacey, 'Body image distortion in non-eating disordered women and men', *Journal of Psychosomatic Research* (1987), 31(4), pp. 513–20, doi:10.1016/0022-3999(87)90009-2.

p. 199 **The technical term for what this question stirs in us is 'functionality appreciation':** J. M. Alleva, T. L. Tylka and A. M. Kroon Van Diest, 'The Functionality Appreciation Scale (FAS): Development and psychometric evaluation in U.S. community women and men', *Body Image* (2017), 23, pp. 28–44, doi:10.1016/j.bodyim.2017.07.008.

p. 199 **when people get out into the natural world, their body image improves significantly:** V. Swami, D. Barron and A. Furnham, 'Exposure to natural environments, and photographs of natural environments, promotes more positive body image', *Body Image* (2018), 24, pp. 82–94.

CHAPTER 10 SELF-ACCEPTANCE V. SELF-STARVATION?

p. 203 **a survey of high school girls found that 50 per cent of them believed they were too fat:** Roberta Pollack Seid, *Never Too Thin: Why Women Are at War with Their Bodies* (Prentice Hall, 1991), p. 150.

p. 206 **She believes that today 'dieting is out, while "elimination" is in':** https://www.stylist.co.uk/long-reads/wellness-ozempic-self-denial/786606, as accessed 3 August 2023.

p. 207 **seems like a type of death:** https://www.stylist.co.uk/long-reads/wellness-ozempic-self-denial/786606, as accessed 3 August 2023.

CHAPTER 11 THE FORBIDDEN BODY?

p. 221 **For people with a BMI higher than 35, it's much worse:** *Oxford Handbook of the Social Science of Obesity*, p. 92; R. M. Puhl et al., 'Perceptions of weight discrimination: prevalence and comparison to race and gender discrimination in America', *International Journal of Obesity (London)* (2008), 32(6), pp. 992–1,000, https://pubmed.ncbi.nlm.nih.gov/18317471/.

p. 222 **women who believed they were overweight, and women who didn't:** B. Major, J. M. Hunger, D. P. Bunyan, and C. T. Miller, 'The ironic effects of weight stigma', *Journal of Experimental Social Psychology* (2014), 51, pp. 74–80, https://doi.org/10.1016/j.jesp.2013.11.009. I learned about this study in K. Gunnars, 'The Harmful Effects of Fat Shaming', *Healthline*, 19 January 2022, https://www.healthline.com/nutrition/fat-shaming-makes-things-worse#overeating.

p. 223 **overweight people who were shown a harsh and judgemental video:** N. A. Schvey et al., 'The impact of weight stigma on caloric consumption', *Obesity (Silver Spring)* (2011), 19(10), pp. 1,957–62, https://pubmed.ncbi.nlm.nih.gov/21760636/ as accessed 10 October 2023.

p. 223 **stigmatising overweight people is in fact counterproductive:** This meta-analysis shows the wider evidence for this: X. Zhu et al., 'A meta-analysis of weight stigma and health behaviors', *Stigma and Health* (2022), 7(1), pp. 1–13, https://doi.org/10.1037/sah0000352; see also A. Tomiyama et al., 'How and why weight stigma drives the obesity "epidemic" and harms health', *BMC Medicine* (2018), 16, p. 123, https://doi.org/10.1186/s12916-018-1116-5.

p. 223 **makes overweight people far less likely to exercise:** L. R. Vartanian et al., 'Effects of Weight Stigma on Exercise Motivation and Behavior: A Preliminary Investigation among College-aged Females', *Journal of Health Psychology* (2008), 13(1), pp. 131–8, https://doi.org/10.1177/1359105307084318.

p. 224 **There is no way to hide being fat except by staying indoors:** Bovey, *Forbidden Body*, p. 1.

p. 224 **A fat man is a joke, and a fat woman is two jokes:** Louise Foxcroft, *Calories and Corsets: A History of Dieting over 2,000 Years* (Profile, 2012), unnumbered opening page.

p. 225 **She also read testimonies from women:** Bovey, *Forbidden Body*, pp. 44–5. **they published a manifesto:** Erec Smith, *Fat Tactics: The Rhetoric and Structure of the Fat Acceptance Movement* (Lexington Books, 2018), pp. 24–5.

p. 227 **one of the first people to warn that obesity had begun to rise:** R. J. Kuczmarski, K. M. Flegal, S. M. Campbell and C. L. Johnson, 'Increasing Prevalence of Overweight Among US Adults: The National Health and Nutrition Examination Surveys, 1960 to 1991', *JAMA* (1994), 272(3), pp. 205–11, doi:10.1001/jama.1994.03520030047027.

p. 227 **she and her colleagues had analysed a dataset of over 36,000 people:** K. M. Flegal et al., 'Excess Deaths Associated With Underweight, Overweight, and Obesity', *JAMA* (2005), 295(15), pp. 1,861–7, https://jamanetwork.com/journals/jama/fullarticle/200731. For Katherine Flegal's perspective on the controversy that followed, see Katherine M. Flegal, 'The obesity wars and the education of a researcher: A personal account', *Progress in Cardiovascular Diseases* (2021), 67, pp. 75–9, https://www.sciencedirect.com/science/article/pii/S0033062021000670.

p. 229 **a small body of scientific research based on a concept called 'Health at Every Size':** See D. Clifford et al., 'Impact of Non-Diet Approaches on Attitudes, Behaviors and Health Outcomes: A Systematic Review', *Journal of Nutrition Education and Behavior* (2015), 47(2), pp. 143–55; L. Bacon and L. Aphramor, 'Weight Science: Evaluating the Evidence for a Paradigm Shift', *Nutrition Journal* (2011), 10(9), https://doi.org/10.1186/1475-2891-10-9; L. Bacon, J. S. Stern, M. D. Van Loan and N. L. Keim, 'Size acceptance and intuitive eating improve health for obese, female chronic dieters', *Journal of the American Dietetic Association* (2005), 105(6), pp. 929–36, doi:10.1016/j.jada.2005.03.011; L. Rapoport, M. Clark and J. Wardle, 'Evaluation of a modified cognitive-behavioural programme for weight management', *International Journal of Obesity and Related Metabolic Disorders* (2000), 24(12), pp. 1,726–37, doi:10.1038/sj.ijo.0801465.

If these approaches really can increase people's exercise levels, they could have a big impact on health – see for example this study (not a 'Health at Every Size' one), which found that an obese person in the 'active' group had half the risk of cardiovascular disease of someone entirely sedentary: X. Zhang et al., 'Physical activity and risk of cardiovascular disease by weight status among US adults', *PLoS One* (2020), 15(5), e0232893, doi:10.1371/journal.pone.0232893.

p. 232 **much more powerful changes than have ever been documented by changes in stress:** Poverty and stress unambiguously do have negative health effects. See for example https://www.thelancet.com/journals/lanepe/

article/PIIS2666-7762(22)00095-3/fulltext. For a discussion of the link between poverty and mortality, see S. Stringhini et al., 'Socioeconomic status and the 25 × 25 risk factors as determinants of premature mortality: a multicohort study and meta-analysis of 1.7 million men and women', *Lancet* (2017), 389(10075), pp. 1,229–37, https://www.thelancet.com/journals/lancet/article/PIIS0140-6736(16)32380-7/fulltext. For a discussion of the link between stress and mortality, see F. Tian et al., 'Association of stress-related disorders with subsequent risk of all-cause and cause-specific mortality: A population-based and sibling-controlled cohort study', *Lancet Regional Health Europe* (2022), 18, https://www.thelancet.com/action/showPdf?pii=S2666-7762%2822%2900095-3.

p. 235 **In response to this critique, Katherine Flegal then did another large-scale study:** K. M. Flegal, B. K. Kit, H. Orpana and B. I. Graubard, 'Association of All-Cause Mortality With Overweight and Obesity Using Standard Body Mass Index Categories: A Systematic Review and Meta-analysis', *JAMA* (2013), 309(1), pp. 71–82, doi:10.1001/jama.2012.113905.

p. 235 **her published data did *not* properly exclude those groups:** He organised a symposium at Harvard where he and several other speakers sought to rebut Flegal's data. See V. Hughes, 'The big fat truth', *Nature* (2013), 497, pp. 428–30, https://doi.org/10.1038/497428a. This piece in Harvard's 'Nutrition Source' blog from 2005 lays out some of Walter's and his colleagues' arguments against Flegal's findings: https://www.hsph.harvard.edu/nutritionsource/2005/05/02/obesity-controversy/.

In 2013 on public radio Walter referred to Flegal's 2013 follow-up study as 'a pile of rubbish'; see 'Shades of grey', *Nature* (2013), 497, p. 410, https://doi.org/10.1038/497410a.

p. 236 **A complex and quite bitter argument over this is still ongoing:** For an excellent summary of that debate, see https://www.theatlantic.com/health/archive/2017/08/is-fat-bad/536652/.

p. 236 **She believes 'we have to deal in reality':** Bovey, *What Have You Got to Lose*, p. 34.

p. 237 **A study by scientists at University College London:** J. Bell et al., 'The Natural Course of Healthy Obesity Over 20 Years', *Journal of the American College of Cardiology* (2015), 65(1), pp. 101–2, https://doi.org/10.1016/j.jacc.2014.09.077. See also Hermann, *Conquering Fat Logic*, p. 83. 'Healthy' and 'unhealthy' had to be very carefully defined in this study. 'Metabolically healthy' they defined as having less than two of the following symptoms: 'high-density lipoprotein cholesterol level <1.03 mmol/l (men) and <1.29 mmol/l (women); blood pressure ≥130/85 mm Hg or use of antihypertensive medication; fasting plasma glucose level ≥5.6 mmol/l or use of antidiabetic medication triacylglycerol level ≥1.7 mmol/l; homeostatic model assessment of insulin resistance >2.87'.

CHAPTER 12 THE LAND THAT DOESN'T NEED OZEMPIC

p. 242 **In July 2023, I stumbled across a curious news story:** 'Slow initial uptake of Novo Nordisk's Wegovy likely in Japan, says analyst', *The Pharma Letter*, 28 July 2023, https://www.thepharmaletter.com/article/slow-initial-uptake-of-novo-nordisk-s-wegovy-likely-in-japan-says-analyst, as accessed 20 September 2023.

p. 242 **Just 3.6 per cent of its people are obese:** N. Yoshiike and M. Miyoshi, 'Epidemiological aspects of overweight and obesity in Japan – international comparisons', *Nihon Rinsho* (2013), 71(2), pp. 207–16, https://pubmed.ncbi.nlm.nih.gov/23631195/#:~:text=Prevalence%20of%20obesity%20(BMI%20%3E%20or,Body%20Mass%20Index%20(WHO), as accessed 20 September 2023.

p. 243 **something happened over a hundred years ago:** Hawaii Health Matters, 'Adults Who Are Obese', https://www.hawaiihealthmatters.org/indicators/index/view?indicatorId=54&localeId=14&localeChartIdxs=1%7C2%7C6, as accessed 15 October 2023. For additional discussion on the comparative health of Japanese Americans and mainland Japanese, see M. Yoneda and K. Kobuke, 'A 50-year history of the health impacts of Westernization on the lifestyle of Japanese Americans: A focus on the Hawaii–Los Angeles–Hiroshima Study', *Journal of Diabetes Investigation* (2020), 11(6), pp. 1,382–7, https://onlinelibrary.wiley.com/doi/full/10.1111/jdi.13278.

p. 247 **we went to the Tokyo College of Sushi and Washoku to interview Masaru Watanabe:** I also interviewed him on Zoom – I have used quotes from both interchangeably here.

p. 264 **Japanese people live longer than anyone else on earth:** S. Tsugane, 'Why has Japan become the world's most long-lived country: insights from a food and nutrition perspective', *European Journal of Clinical Nutrition* (2021), 75, pp. 921–8, https://doi.org/10.1038/s41430-020-0677-5.

p. 264 **The average American and British person is in poor health:** 'Healthy life expectancy (HALE) at birth (years)', Global Health Observatory, World Health Organization, 12 April 2020, https://www.who.int/data/gho/data/indicators/indicator-details/GHO/gho-ghe-hale-healthy-life-expectancy-at-birth, as accessed 26 October 2023.

p. 264 **In Japan, it's five to six years:** See Table 1 in S. Tsugane, 'Why has Japan become the world's most long-lived country' pp. 921–8, https://doi.org/10.1038/s41430-020-0677-5. See also S. Tokudome, A. Igata and S. Hashimoto, 'Life expectancy and healthy life expectancy of Japan: the fastest graying society in the world', *BMC Research Notes* (2016), 9, pp. 1–6.

p. 264 **in Japan, it's just one in thirty-eight:** 'Breast Cancer Rates Rising Among Japanese Women', Roswell Park Comprehensive Cancer Center, 25 July 2017, https://www.roswellpark.org/cancertalk/201707/breast-cancer-rates-rising-among-japanese-women#:~:text=%E2%80%9CIn%20 general%2C%201%20out%20of,Roswell%20Park%20Comprehens ive%20Cancer%20Center, as accessed 1 October 2023.

p. 265 **It has 215 households, and 173 people there are ninety or older:** I was given these numbers by Fumiaru Osaki, who works in the nearby tourist office, and consulted the official Japanese census figures for me. I got the idea to go to Ogimi after reading about it in Booth, *Sushi and Beyond*, pp. 267–81.

p. 269 **In most places where this has been tried, it has reduced purchases of these drinks:** One review of studies estimated that purchases and consumption of sugary drinks drop by 10 per cent with each 10 per cent increase in taxes. See A. M. Teng et al., 'Impact of sugar-sweetened beverage taxes on purchases and dietary intake: Systematic review and meta-analysis', *Obesity Reviews* (2019), 20(9), pp. 1,187–204, https://onlinelibrary.wiley.com/doi/10.1111/obr.12868. See also https://www.ncbi.nlm.nih.gov/pmc/articles/PMC5525113/.

p. 270 **In just four years, they cut childhood obesity:** Warner, *The Truth About Fat*, p. 323; S. Boseley, 'Amsterdam's solution to the obesity crisis: no fruit juice and enough sleep', *Guardian*, 14 April 2017, https://www.theguardian.com/society/2017/apr/14/amsterdam-solution-obes ity-crisis-no-fruit-juice-enough-sleep, as accessed 12 October 2023. See also UNICEF, City of Amsterdam and EAT, 'The Amsterdam Healthy Weight Approach: Investing in healthy urban childhoods: A case study on healthy diets for children', 2020, https://www.unicef.org/media/89401/file/Amsterdam-Healthy-Weight-Approach-Investing-healthy-urban-childhoods.pdf, as accessed 12 October 2023. I also consulted the report by NJi, VU University Amsterdam and Cuprifère Consult, 'Amsterdam Approach to Healthy Weight: promising? A search for the active elements', https://npo.nl/npo3/brandpuntplus/hoe-een-wethouder-afrekende-met-obesitas-in-zijn-stad, as accessed 12 October 2023. Thank you to Rosanne Kropman for translating.

p. 270 **A study showed that after six months, her patients felt significantly healthier:** S. Kempainen et al., 'A Collaborative Pilot to Support Patients With Diabetes Through Tailored Food Box Home Delivery', *Health Promotion Practice* (2023), 24(5), pp. 963–8, doi:10.1177/15248399221100792.

p. 270 **It saves between 6,000 and 9,000 lives a year from strokes in the UK alone:** J. Song et al., 'Salt intake, blood pressure and cardiovascular disease mortality in England, 2003–2018', *Journal of Hypertension* (November 2023), doi: 10.1097/HJH.0000000000003521. See also https://journals.lww.com/jhypertension/fulltext/2023/11000/salt_intake,_blood_pres sure_and_cardiovascular.6.aspx https://www.qmul.ac.uk/wiph/news/lat est-news/items/increased-salt-intake-in-england-from-2014-18.html, as accessed 25 November 2023.

p. 271 **It increased life expectancy in the North Karelia region, where these changes began, by ten years, and by seven years in the rest of Finland:**

V. Salomaa et al., 'Decline of coronary heart disease mortality in Finland during 1983 to 1992: roles of incidence, recurrence, and case-fatality. The FINMONICA MI Register Study', *Circulation* (1996), 94(12), pp. 3,130–7, doi:10.1161/01.cir.94.12.3130; P. Puska and P. Jaini, 'The North Karelia Project: Prevention of Cardiovascular Disease in Finland Through Population-Based Lifestyle Interventions', *American Journal of Lifestyle Medicine* (2020), 14(5), pp. 495–9, https://pubmed.ncbi.nlm.nih.gov/32922234/. As reported in the latter paper, the death rate from cardiovascular disease in North Karelia reduced from 690 per 100,000 in the 1960s to 100 per 100,000 in 2011; that's less than half the current USA rate of 209 per 100,000. See https://www.cdc.gov/nchs/fastats/heart-disease.htm, as accessed 24 November 2023.

p. 278 **the number of obese kids in Britain shot up by 70 per cent:** Shell, *The Hungry Gene*, p. 3.

p. 278 **the rate of increase in childhood obesity doubled during the pandemic years:** O. Dyer, 'Obesity in US children increased at an unprecedented rate during the pandemic', *BMJ* (2021), 374, n2332, https://www.bmj.com/content/374/bmj.n2332, as accessed 21 September 2023.

p. 278 **consumed by kids in the US come from ultra-processed foods:** L. Wang et al., 'Trends in Consumption of Ultraprocessed Foods Among US Youths Aged 2–19 Years, 1999–2018', *JAMA* (2021), 326(6), pp. 519–30, doi:10.1001/jama.2021.10238. I first learned about this figure in Tim Spector, *Food For Life* (Jonathan Cape, 2022), p. 36.

p. 278 **A summary of the evidence was published in *Pediatrics*:** S. Hampl et al., 'Clinical Practice Guideline for the Evaluation and Treatment of Children and Adolescents With Obesity', *Pediatrics* (2023), 151, 2, e2022060640, https://doi.org/10.1542/peds.2022-060640.

p. 278 **The largest clinical trial on young people:** D. Weghuber et al., 'Once-Weekly Semaglutide in Adolescents with Obesity', *New England Journal of Medicine* (2022), 387(24), pp. 2,245–57, doi:10.1056/NEJMoa2208601. Sixty-two of the kids in the trial were just given a placebo, and they aren't included in the 131 figure given. See also https://www.theguardian.com/society/2023/may/17/half-of-children-given-skinny-jab-no-longer-clinically-obese-us-study, as accessed 24 November 2023.

p. 279 **Dan Cooper, a professor of paediatrics at the University of California, Irvine:** https://www.cambridge.org/core/journals/journal-of-clinical-and-translational-science/article/unintended-consequences-of-glucagonlike-peptide1-receptor-agonists-medications-in-children-and-adolescents-a-call-to-action/F0286F2FBBD7F6E4E75A6A383F3C82BB.

p. 283 **This is not because of the inherent cost of these drugs:** J. Levi et al., 'Estimated minimum prices and lowest available national prices for antiobesity medications: Improving affordability and access to treatment', *Obesity (Silver Spring)* (2023), 31, pp. 1,270–9, https://doi.org/10.1002/oby.23725, as accessed 10 October 2023.

INDEX